Meribeth Bunch Dayme

Dynamics of the Singing Voice

Fifth Edition

SpringerWienNewYork

Meribeth Bunch Dayme, Ph.D.
Consultant in Voice, London, England

With illustrations by Audrey Besterman
Consultant for Anatomical Portions: Ruth E.M. Bowden

© 2009 Springer-Verlag/Wien
Printed in Austria
Springer-Verlag Wien New York is a part of
Springer Science + Business Media
springer.at

Typesetting and Printing: Holzhausen Druck & Medien GmbH, 1140 Vienna, Austria

Printed on acid-free and chlorine-free bleached paper
SPIN: 12463329

With 67 Figures

Library of Congress Control Number: 2009927288

ISBN 978-3-211-88728-8 SpringerWienNewYork
ISBN 3-211-82985-7 4th edn. SpringerWienNewYork

Foreword

This 5th Edition of Dynamics of the Singing Voice represents an amalgamation of the new and the old. The most dramatic changes are the first four chapters, which point to many possible new directions in this century. The sections on vocal anatomy have only minor changes because the anatomy has not changed. Our understanding of function has evolved, but as of yet, not as much as we would like. For this reason, a Chapter 12, Research in Singing was written.

The advent of the Internet brought the world to everyone, as almost anything you want to know can be found there. It is easy to be a scholar now—just ask any of the search engines. For this reason, the old, vast bibliography has been updated and trimmed. When the original book was written, there were no comprehensive bibliographies for singers to study and it was done as a service. Now there are so many excellent texts with huge numbers of references by Sataloff, Titze, Sundberg, and many others.

As a help to all those singers who struggle with the science and anatomy, Study Outlines for Vocal Anatomy have been included in the appendices. These were originally written for my vocal anatomy courses.

The book emphasizes vocal anatomy with little attention being given to acoustics. There are excellent treatices on acoustics by Titze, Sundberg, Howard and others who know far more than I in this area.

Over the years of the publication of this book, much has changed; and that includes the author. I apologize if the writing style is slightly different in the new and old sections. The study of the human voice, and now energy field, has been a source of never ending fascination for me. I wish the same for you in your pursuit of singing and teaching.

Preface

The end is now the beginning

When Dynamics of the Singing Voice was written more than twenty-five years ago, it answered a need to know. This new edition is about the need to understand. As Einstein stated so aptly: *A man should look for what is, and not for what he thinks should be. Information is not knowledge.*

The aim of this new edition is to look at ways we can expand our knowledge by looking for what is, and explore new frontiers in voice and singing while at the same time honoring what we have from the past. The understanding of the physical structure, psychology, and old pedagogical methods are no longer sufficient and we need to spend time evaluating what is and was useful, and what no longer serves us. Not only has science expanded enormously and taken great leaps, so has our understanding of the whole world of self-development--physically, mentally and spiritually. It is time for us to look at these developments in relation to the human voice and to the teaching of singing.

Our intellectual knowledge of the voice has increased multifold over the past thirty years and will continue. However, this is only one side of a very incomplete picture. The need to satisfy academic guidelines, and quantify information in order to prove its value, has made us overly analytical/critical in areas where we have no need for those kinds of conversations, inner or outer, and has upset the balance of how we learn, teach, and perform.

The previous editions of this book emphasized the need to understand the physical structure of the vocal mechanism and to be able to communicate this. Certainly, this is now part of most graduate curricula in vocal pedagogy, and while it is still important to know this information, it no longer is necessary to emphasize it to the detriment of seeing the larger context. This edition of *Dynamics of the Singing Voice* retains much of its original information on vocal anatomy with the exception of small alterations throughout. Students and teachers all over the world have loved the clarity of the writing about the anatomy, so I would not change that. Study quides I created for my vocal anatomy courses also have been added as appendices to help you learn. You will note that while the physical aspects of voice still occupy most of the space in the book, they are now located at the end because concepts being explored in the last chapters of previous editions are very important to what is happening now. In the last thirty-five years there has been huge expansion of knowledge and information relating to areas of self-development, quantum concepts in science and healing, and access to singing, sounds and music from every corner of the world.

Scientists, especially the quantum physicists, no longer speak of the human body as being composed of molecules or atoms; it is now the human energy field, the fabric of the universe, and particles (and lately strings). We will take a look at these expanded concepts and how they change the emphasis from the physical structure, to the broader areas of our thinking, teaching, relationships, therapy, and performance. We are beginning to see the merging of the arts, sciences, self-development, and spirituality in exciting ways that are meaningful to voice professionals. These ideas are now explored in the opening chapters along with the implications for a new look at vocal pedagogy, and practical ways of implementing these concepts in teaching and performing in the 21st Century.

This current edition is a compilation of years of my own growth and development, teaching and experience, as well as the thinking, ideas, and creativity of many. The feedback and appreciation of students and teachers who have studied and taught this text over the years has been gratifying. As I have learned from everyone, it would be impossible to name all the students, teachers and colleagues who have directly or indirectly contributed to the ideas contained in these pages. However, I must express my gratitude for the wise teaching and hours of enlightening discussion with several people who are now with us in spirit only, the late William Vennard, a singer and teacher of distinction, a close musical friend, Shibley Boyes, and Professor R.V. Gregg who first taught me anatomy.

Without the skilled correction, discussion and editorial contribution of the late Professor R. E. M. Bowden relating to anatomy, this book would not have had the same quality. Not only did she give of her profound knowledge of anatomy, which she taught at The Royal Free Hospital School of Medicine and The Royal College of Surgeons for many, many years, but also her excellent literary skills. For all that I am deeply grateful. My thanks also to Audrey Besterman, a superb medical illustrator, the photographic departments of the Royal College of Surgeons, the Royal Free Hospital School of Medicine and the Institute of Neurology; and to these institutions for giving me bench space and help with my original work; to Rita Farrell for her guidance and work on the early stages of the original manuscript; to Gloria Prosper who contributed to the early formation of the extensive Bibliography; and to the National Institutes of Health for the post doctoral research grant which made it possible for me to find the time to further my own research and to write the first edition of this book.

Recently, my own career in the arts, science, business, healing, and spirituality led me to look for a way to bring my various *hats* under one large umbrella. Often we find what we are searching for in places where we are not looking, and this happened to me. As fate would have it, I attended an intriguing course on energetic healing taught by Louise Mita. Thus began the understanding of how all my hats could, and have, fit under the umbrella of energy work. Energy work and healing have strengthened and encompassed every aspect of my previous study, enlarged my already great curiosity, and sent me on a journey to find out even more. The excitement of learning, growing, and of sharing this knowledge is part of my mission to help singers, their teachers, and professionals who work with singers. For this added energy and joy of new adventure at this time in my life, I thank you, Louise Mita. Finally, I express my profound gratitude to Jane Vukovic for her support in every way over the past thirty years.

January 2009, Lake Annecy, France   *Meribeth Dayme, PhD*

Contents

Contents

Introduction 1

Core singing

New approaches to singing for the 21st Century

The first edition of this book mainly addressed how the voice functions based on what we knew at that time. It ended with a discussion of how the rather large amount of published material relating Eastern and Western philosophies to sound and singing might be considered in the future. That future time has arrived faster than any of us could have imagined and the final chapter of Dynamics of the Singing Voice, editions 1-4, now forms part of this Introduction. Here is how it was stated in previous editions.

As singing and singers evolve they will not be able to ignore the importance and impact of current and future knowledge of Eastern and Western philosophies, because it will enable performers to achieve a wholeness that contributes significantly to the tangible and intangible qualities of sound. How a person relates to him/herself and achieves wholeness is an important aspect of singing and there are a number of areas along these lines which merit study: physical factors at macro and micro-levels, vibration, "quantum" factors, sound and healing and purity of emotions. These factors are an important part of the vitality and "life energy' of the singer and of the resulting power of the music presented. Healthy energy in the singer creates the same in the audience, whereas poor energy can leave the listener feeling down or drained for no apparent reason (Diamond, 1983). Ideally, the listener will leave feeling energised and enhanced. In the past singers have tended to be more concerned with the voice rather than the actual effect it was having, the actual making of the tone and the science of it, getting involved emotionally without allowing the audience to feel for themselves, and generally missing out on true listening and awareness of self, audience and the atmosphere. When singers begin to incorporate a wider awareness of these things in a positive manner the sound of the future will come from the 'spirit' and the heart rather than an obsession with my voice and my tone.

The earlier work in the 80's and 90's around life energy by Diamond, in quantum healing by Chopra, in the Tao and physics by Capra, and so many others, has expanded into the fields of learning, teaching, healing, and self-development so fast, and with so many derivations and new investigations, that we are experiencing a whole new wave of information propelling us into the 21st Century. The field of singing and the voice must stay in touch and in tune with this because it will change singing and how we work with singers for years to come.

Capra (1990) and Greene (2003) in physics, Pert (1997) and Taylor (2008) in physiology, and Chopra (1989) and Hunt (1996) in energy and healing introduced the layperson to new and fascinating aspects of quantum physics, physiology, and healing that describe smaller and smaller units of energy. These units permeate and pervade everything that exists to form the constitution of space itself. (The physicists refer to it as the *fabric of the universe or matrix*). Therefore everything, including man, his thoughts, actions and movements, is part of the whole; every single thought and event affecting everything else. It is interesting to consider how this differs little from sound, which travels in invisible, but audible, waves filling space and furnishing energy to an arena or auditorium full of people. Performer and audience have an effect on each other. It is essential that singers and teachers now become aware of the need to learn about the affects of energy and how to use it wisely and responsibly in performance and teaching.

Core singing[1] uses the knowledge and understanding of all the aspects of the energy field to develop personally, musically and artistically from the commencement of study to performance. This book will look at ways this understanding can be brought to singers and those professionals who work with them.

What are some of the key issues that need to be addressed today? What major areas around singing and the teaching of singing are causing singers to fall behind other professions that involve performance? What follows is a description of five of the key issues relating to learning, the language of the mind, developing the innate or natural talent that is there, overcoming performance anxiety, and looking beyond the narrow confines of the teaching and research in our own field to learn from others. These issues will be addressed in subsequent chapters in more detail. How we develop as teachers and singers is an important part of the new learning and teaching. Singers and voice professionals

---

[1] While this text is directed towards singing, the author considers the information regarding 'singing' applicable to the production of human vocal sound whether it is sung or spoken.

need ways to deal with a world that is moving so fast that change is happening in months and not years. How can we help them to do that?

Key issues in singing today

While those performers and athletes whose professional life depends on peak performance are quick to utilise techniques that are derived from Eastern and Western philosophies and practices, those in the field of voice and singing have been somewhat reluctant to follow. The "collective consciousness" of several hundred years of the formal teaching of singing has been slow to embrace mind-body concepts such as Alexander Technique, Feldenkrais, Yoga, meditation, alternative therapies, healing martial arts forms such as Qigong, and other variations of these systems. There has been a reluctance to enjoy pursuing the unknown as the quantum physicists and other scientists now have to do on a daily basis. According to Lipton (2005), *today's scientist is finding that by giving the energy-based environment its due, it provides the foundation for the science and philosophy of complementary medicine and the spiritual wisdom of ancient and modern faiths as well as for allopathic medicine.* Singing is not something outside of this energy-based environment; it is directly in the middle.

The following five areas are crucial to the further evolution of singing and the teaching of singing.

a) The approach to teaching and learning

Because there has not been a clear understanding that all of our various levels of energy are connected, it is easy to see why teaching and vocal research has been unknowingly limited to a small part of the singer's energy field. Rarely does a teacher or voice professional address the whole person. The perception is that time does not permit it. Yet, there is every possibility that a more informed approach greatly would improve the efficiency of learning and/or therapy. It has not been fully comprehended that language, thoughts, emotions, and perceptions affect and influence everyone. The language of teaching is powerful and contributes significantly to the inner talk, language, and confidence of the student. This can answer the strange issue as to why singers sometimes feel they sing better at home than in a lesson. Perhaps they are not expected to sing well by the teacher, or show improvement to the therapist. And, unless singers are extremely powerful and confident, they then duly live out these unconscious expectations and develop fear. Current teaching and therapy are full of language, said or unsaid, often unintentional, that leaves a negative impression on the energy field and inhibits the amount that can be achieved in a lesson or performance. As Michael Phelps said after winning his eighth gold medal: *"Nothing is impossible. With so many people saying it couldn't be done, all it takes is an imagination, and that's something I learned and something that helped me."* This is what singers need to learn as well.

b) The language of the mind

The language learned from parents, relatives, teachers, and peers contributes both to personal mind chatter, or the inner voice, and how we speak to others. Our educational systems encourage students to be analytical/critical in their academic studies. However, important this might be for the development of the intellect, it is not necessarily a useful practice in self-development or in developing the awareness and centeredness needed for performance. According to Taylor (2008), all the language, ego, emotional baggage we keep repeating, memory of past events, rote learning, and more, are housed in the left-brain in a group of cells that occupy the space of a peanut. It is really not a good idea for this tiny "peanut' to rule learning, teaching and the development of a singer—or any other performer. The intuitive, sensitive, full awareness that comes with use of the right brain is necessary for optimum performance. For example, a singer can learn words by rote and endless repetition, but this only stores the information in the left-brain—and can be easily forgot in the nervousness of performance. When the same singer learns the words by creating pictures, movements, colours, immediately the text is part of a much larger portion of the energy field and the singer is less likely to have issues with remembering the words—or their imagination. Currently singers and teachers are confusing left-brain information with true knowledge and awareness (right-brain). Balance needs to be restored in our approach to teaching and learning.

The result of an overly analytical/critical approach is singers who have a constant conversation, usually critical, going on in their heads at the time they need to be in a performance state, sometimes referred to as the zone by athletes. This criticism embeds itself in the energy field around the singer and creates blockages to efficient learning and effective performance. When this happens, there is no way of knowing just how much talent or potential a performer really can demonstrate.

The possibilities today for developing the balanced performer are unlimited. With the accessibility of courses and therapies from every tradition, East, West, and mixtures of the both, to new creative, helpful therapies happening in the area of energy healing and medicine, there is little excuse not to find a way to develop the potential that we all have. It is a normal part of the development of world-class athletes to use these systems to reach their performance potential. Singers can do this too.

c) Developing talent

How we develop and encourage the talents of potential singers is changing rapidly at this time. The concepts of the "traditional teaching" of singing are being re-assessed in a number of ways. First, the "pure classical" tradition has been eroded by the success of contemporary commercial and world music. World wide media via television and the Internet furnish and expose us to an infinite variety of sounds, and multi-cultural traditions of singing that were not available in the same way twenty-five years ago. This exposure has given us new vocal colours and unlimited possibilities of sound to explore in the singing voice. These sounds are in the ear of singers today, and are having a conscious and subconscious influence whether we like it or not.

Second, the question now is more "Is the voice healthy, rather than is it "correct"—because what is correct differs greatly in each genre and style. The idea that only certain sounds are healthy has been severely challenged by hearing perfectly healthy singing in everything from multi-tonal music such as overtone chanting, the gutteral and raspy sounds heard in African singing, and some contemporary singers who use it deliberately, and the infinite possibilities of sound taken from combinations of various cultural and classical styles.

When these singing styles and traditions do not create vocal pathology in the singer, then the voice can be deemed healthy. It becomes a matter of taste and choice for the singer and the listener. The concentration then moves to the education of performers who are able to handle variety, open to new sounds and expressions, and are responsible enough to make wise choices for their voices. This will happen when singers are fully in touch with themselves, and the music at the same time. Self-development, discipline, and dedication to the technique and the music all help ground singers and change fear of performance to excitement, passion, and communicating their love of the music to the audience.

d) Learning to trust the voice

Too many singers/performers are unable to share their love and excitement because they do not trust themselves or their voices. While performance anxiety has been researched at length, the symptoms rather than the causes have been addressed. Beta-blockers and other medications and drugs may dull the effect of fear. However until the issues of how fear develops are addressed, it will be difficult to have confident, centred performers.

What are some of the possible causes of fear in performance? First, singers rarely decide for themselves how something sounds. Traditionally, a teacher or coach will tell them when it is correct, and singers are then left to find that sound again, once they are on their own. It is difficult to trust your voice when you are always dependent on someone else to verify the sound for you. While expert guidance is necessary, the singer needs to have co-responsibility for the lesson and the vocal end result. The singers, teachers and therapists who make use of a video in lessons have far better results in the long term. Singers can see for themselves why something is successful or not because it is not left to trial and error or accident. Audio feedback is useful, but it is not as effective as video because it does not allow the performer to experience the total communication package of the visual, vocal and textual at the same time.

The traditional language of right versus wrong, and an analytical/critical approach increase fear as well. Above all, singers need to value their own voice and appreciate the fact that they are singers regardless of their standing in the profession. When singers are taught to be grateful, rather than always critical for the sounds they produce, and at the same time to be disciplined in approach and technique, dedicated to study, and encouraged to be imaginative and creative, then fear will not a part of the picture. There will not be a question of whether the "right" sound is being produced. Singing will be part of the whole of the performance. With a different use of language, techniques of self-development and healing, singers have the potential to be far more efficient now and in the future. Gratitude and love of the art will replace fear and give us skilled performers who are dedicated to the mission of singing.

e) Awareness and responsibility

The media in its various forms offers singers and teachers so many options that it can confuse the neophyte and dull the senses of the wider audience to quality. While the media represents a veritable cornucopia of treasures from television to Internet, to computer software that allows recording and karaoke, it offers at the same time every variation of quality. There is even more reason for the singer to know what he or she wants and be able to make informed decisions. Ideally the decision making process would include feedback, information and advice from the voice professional combined with the sensibility of the singer.

The teacher is responsible for being able to offer options, and think "outside the box" when necessary to help singers develop their innate talent to the best of their ability. Not all students will become professional performers, however, they will add a very satisfying skill that honours their creativity and enhances their wellbeing. Singing lifts the spirit and has long been a part of every culture. Those who sing to and for themselves are generally happy people.

Students are responsible for being aware of their own energy field, maintaining a healthy, helpful inner voice, learning a healthy technique, having the courage to take creative risks, and to know when singing is the real mission they have in this life.

"Will the person eager to perform a creative act serve, in the name of self expression, the wants of his or her ego-dominated and culturally determined personality – or will the activity be performed in the service of humanity beyond socio-cultural attachments and expectations of results, as a humble and transpersonal attempt to do what one simply has to do, because it is one's dharma, the central truth of one's being?
Every issue in the world of music and the arts, around which arguments rage and coteries are formed extolling this or that procedure, can be reformulated in terms of this central question. The answer is given by the quality of being the creative activity radiates and the character and scope of the consistent and sustained meaning that infuses and empowers the activity." (Rudhyar, 1982).

The quote above is the challenge for the singer of the 21st Century to go beyond. This means performing with a proper sense of detachment, warmth, no interference by the ego, being completely in phase with the pulse of the music, being centred, loving what he or she is doing and communicating that love.

What can only follow is a performance that is positive, vibrant, with the power to heal both singer and audience. *"But the human sender … is also his own receiver. An artist constantly communicates with his growing work of art. As the work grows, its communicative power imbues the artist as much as the artist gives to the work"* (Clynes, 1989).

The question remains: will the singer sing? Or be sung?

2 The human energy field and singing

Defining the human energy field

Singers live with the feelings of the vibration of their own voices on an everyday basis and it is easy for them to embrace the concept that energy or vibration is basic to everything that exists. Eastern and Western cultures describe it in different ways. Biologists see energy as part of human life such as breath and pulse, physicists as quantum particles, and spiritual traditions speak of *prana, chi* (Qi) and light. The importance of energy is recognized in medicine and various health professions by the use of therapeutic and diagnostic tools such as ultrasound, electric pulse, shock wave therapy, and magnetic resonance imaging to name a few (See Oschman, 2000). In the field of complementary and alternative medicine energy healing comes in many forms: from hands-on work, natural energies like crystals and magnets, acupuncture, life force or chi, to radionics and mind. These are being used to great effect—some prominent examples being: various forms of kinesiology such as Edu-K™, EFT (Emotional Freedom Technique™) and Quantum Touch™ (See Gordon (2006), Feinstein and Eden (2005), and Integrative Quantum Medicine™ (Mita, taoenergy.com). These and other therapies will be discussed more fully in Chapter 11 on Vocal Health.

As reported by Braden (2007), *"Scientists believe that more than ninety percent of the cosmos is invisible to our eyes and appears to us as empty space This energy seems to be everywhere, always, and to have existed since the very beginning of time more"*. We are aware of energies we cannot see such as gravity, because we work with them all the time. In reality, what we call *space* is not empty at all; it is occupied by a dynamic field of invisible particles. The human body, a dense quantum field, becomes a small part of the whole picture in relation to the vast amount of space that is perceived as empty.

Diamond (1983) defined 'life energy' as being a vital force that is physical, mental and spiritual in nature: the physical being reflected in muscular activity and the functioning of the skeletal system; the mental including thoughts and the ability to be centered; and the spiritual that begins as spirit which is signified by the love and humanity within each person. He has also noted that everything in the environment, both physical and psychic – thoughts, feelings, desires, etc. – affects life energy.

Life energy is only one part of a quantum energy field that includes every kind of imaginable energy from the sun, earth, wind, the human life force, to mind power. Energies are usually divided into three major categories: 1. The basic physical, earth, and minute quantum energies such as solar, magnetism, gravity, nuclear, radiation, fire, wind and so on; 2. life force energies that include the Eastern concept of Qi or chi (each culture has different words for this, i.e. prana in India), acupuncture meridians, and the chakra system described in Eastern practices and now widespread in Western alternative healing techniques; 3. the most powerful of all, the mind (Xen or Shen for the Chinese) and spiritual energy. Therefore in view of the information and knowledge explosion we are currently experiencing, the mechanics of singing need to be regarded in a new light.

Components of the human energy field

Contemporary scientists doing research in energy generally include some or all of the following aspects when describing the human energy field: the physical, metaphysical, mental, emotional, psychological, psychic and spiritual. (See Hunt, 1996; Lipton, 2005). Traditional Chinese Medicine uses similar components, but combines these in different ways.

The most obvious components of the energy field are the human body and our visible physical surroundings. To learn that the body and what we see is less than ten percent of the whole is daunting. How is it that we have missed so much? One reason is that our analytical/critical bias has insisted that we look at only those things that we could see, or that offered sufficient statistical proof. The empirical studies often have been discounted. This is why traditions and practices that have existed, and been successful, for thousands of years have been given short shrift in contemporary practice until recently. The systems of proof available to most of the Western world are mainly those that satisfy the "peanut sized cell area" in the left-brain. The left-brain is also the source of the ego that has a difficult time giving up old, or potentially threatening concepts. The quantum physicists have been the scientists who have had to venture into the world of the unseen, without expectations. They are leading the way in the current thinking that is guiding work in biology, chemistry, medicine, physics and energy healing.

What are some of the major components of the invisible energy that affect everything about how we sing, perform, and control our lives. The visible physical area is the last place that energy imbalances show themselves. So much has to have happened before we are aware of physical symptoms.

Invisible aspects of the energy field

Teachers and therapists know that they can have a physically perfect person in front of them and yet that person cannot sing well. To continue to look for physical or acoustic reasons would just be a waste of time. Something else needs attention or is missing. There are a number of areas to begin the search.

a) Mental aspects

Mental preparation for singing, whether practice or performance, is a key ingredient in providing a healthy energy field for singing. Attitude and motivation are key ingredients in singing and a quiet mind and mental discipline are paths to the healthy thinking needed for performance. Negative thoughts, stress, past traumas relating to performance or lessons, busy mind chatter while singing, trying to remember the words, and everything the teacher said, create a mind that is too busy to sing and cause low energy on the part of the singer. When singers are busy anticipating problems, they are likely to get rewarded with what they fear most. Audiences consciously or subconsciously pick up negative or low energy, which is unhealthy; and they go away dissatisfied without knowing why. Therefore it is up to the individual singer to make sure that he is focused on being fully present.

An old Eastern description of being centered includes the analogy of the wheel. While a wheel has many spokes, it the empty center that enables it to go around. Perhaps this is the most difficult thing in singing because it means having the discipline and persistence to know the words, and music well, and at the same time the ability to be centered and in touch with intuition, imagination and the quiet inner self during the performance. "*We intuitively distinguish a genuine, deeply felt communication from superficial expressions ... to pay attention to these ... involves an intense quietness, a true listening*" (Clynes, 1979). Each person has to find his or her own way of centering and there are many Eastern and Western spiritual, religious and ethical methods, philosophies, and books which teach this skill and make it available to anyone interested. It is beyond the scope of this book to discuss specific exercises and disciplines related to centering, however many of these 'paths' talk about silence within silence, being still and remaining detached. The singer can achieve this with guidance and practice. The result is a singer who can imagine and expect to enjoy performing and give his best to the audience. The goal of being able to listen and sense what is happening in performance without interfering mentally, emotionally or musically is necessary for optimum performance.

b) Emotions

Emotions can heal, or create chaos with the energy field. Contemporary scientists and medical practitioners from Eastern and Western cultures are finding common physiological and philosophical concepts of the body/mind in relation to emotion. Pert (1997), Chia (2005), and Taylor (2008) are examples of three contemporary voices on the subject.

"According to Chinese medicine, there is no single headquarters in the brain that regulates mood and emotion. Rather the receptors and transmitters that relate to mood and emotion are dispersed throughout the body and brain. The energetic meridians in the body are multi-dimensional and create a functional interaction between the body/mind/emotions and the universe. These energetic patterns affect the body, personality, character, mood, and emotional attributes.
The Chinese understanding of mood and emotion is organic and holistic.....stress arises as a reaction resulting from desire. If there is no desire, the mood is stable. Persistent negative emotions alter the bodily condition, as the organs can no longer regulate and balance each other. Somatic disorders and psychosomatic symptoms appear as stressful characteristics in the body/mind." (Chia 2005)

Pert (1997) is known for her research on neurotransmitters and their effect on mood. *"The immune cells are making the same chemicals that we conceive of as controlling mood in the brain. So immune cells not only control the tissue integrity of the body, but they also manufacture information chemicals that can regulate mood or emotion... We can no longer think of the emotions as having less validity than physical, material substance, but instead must see them as cellular signals that are involved in the process of translating information into physical reality; literally transforming mind into matter."*

According to Taylor (2008), a neuroscientist, it takes ninety seconds for an emotion to transit the body physiologically. If we could then get that emotion, or what created it, out of our mind, we would be clear. However, every time we remember the event, or repeat it, we bring back the physiological experience of that emotion. For example every time people replay past angry or fearful scenes in their minds, they recreate the same physiological reaction as the original scene and stress organs and the immune system in the process.

People imprint stress and negative feelings on their energy field by the constant repetition. This has a domino effect at every level until it reaches the physical, where some sort of pathology can be the negative result.

Emotion in singing is a topic that usually is ignored or omitted because it is difficult to quantify. However, Dr. Manfred Clynes (1989) in his book, *Sentics: The Touch of the Emotions,* has gone a long way towards clarifying and defining what pure emotion means because he has found a way to measure and quantify the pure states of joy, love, grief, hate, anger and no emotion. His discussion about the communication of emotion deserves the attention of every singer.

Clynes explains that *"the power of sentic [emotional] form to generate sentic states in the perceiver is greatly dependent upon its purity."* He defines purity of emotion as the degree to which it approximates or is faithful to the inner emotional form. *"By being open to being 'used by the source of purity', we may be enabled to communicate it, becoming its vessels* – one way of describing performing or singing naturally.

Performing naturally means two things: (1) to listen inwardly with utmost precision to the inner form of every musical sound, and (2) then to produce that form precisely. It means to have a precise idea, as well as a precise execution of it. And the crucial and amazing fact is that if one really believes this and listens with great care, then it also turns out to be beautiful." (Clynes, 1989).

For the performer to be able to listen in this way, demands complete detachment; almost that of a meditative state or that of a third person viewing from the outside. As the 'observer', the singer can then allow the music to tell its own story without interference because *"simultaneous production and perception of the same emotional form cannot be carried out by the nervous system without a degree of interference."*

The pure emotional form induces empathy and is experienced as 'sincerity' by the listener. *"This empathy arises when, in the manifest openness of the person expressing, we sense that the expression arises from the centre of his being ..."* What the singer often perceives when learning this detachment and purity is a sense of being out of control and not having enough color and expression. The temptation is to do more because it feels as it nothing is happening. Learning to overcome those feelings and the temptation to meddle is an important part of becoming an artist who is performing from the heart rather than the head.

c) Psychological influences

Psychological aspects include: self-esteem, overcoming limitations and dealing with the ego. Self-esteem is an important part of a singer's repertoire. Some performers are not sure of the difference between self-esteem and ego. The ego is a product of some of the endless repetition and mind-chatter of the left-brain (See Tolle, 2005, and Taylor, 2008). Self-esteem is an inner sense of worth without the need for the rest of the world to know about it.

A healthy psychological aspect of a singer's energy field includes the ability to overcome limitations imposed from the self, family, friends, colleagues and teachers. There are many gifted singers who come from a non-musical family tradition. As the first in the family, they often get overloaded with the family belief that "no-one in that family is musical, or able to become professional, or you cannot make any money from singing. Overcoming these constant thoughts and statements, becomes a challenge. The weak person will give in and adopt these negative beliefs and lose self-esteem.

d) Psychic aspects

Part of the psychic energy of every singer is the collective mind or consciousness built up over several hundred years about singing and how it is taught. This invisible aspect of energy is like a huge collection of thoughts and customs and plays a large part in singing. While there is something to be said for tradition, it is also good to be able to get outside and look in where the past is concerned. The argument stated by people who are caught up in the psychic web of collective consciousness is: "everyone does it this way". Learning from the collective wisdom is important; blindly accepting the collective folly is not very useful. When teachers and students are taught in such a way that they can see for themselves and take equal responsibility for learning, then the inner wisdom of each person will guide the discoveries that are to be made rather than the need to conform to a lesser quality.

Many singers have used drugs to give themselves psychic experiences that they believe enhance performance. They also have taken drugs

to avoid nerves and performance anxiety. The perception of the feeling
and the result are not compatible. Singers who do this most often fool
themselves, and not the audience. The *zone* that they want is one of inner quietude and a co-ordination of all the elements of the energy field.
Athletes are taught to reach this through visualization and meditation.
When singers make this a part of their preparation for performance, lessons and auditions, they will be able to find the *zone* without help from
drugs or alcohol.

e) Spiritual aspects

The moment a singer is free enough to allow his spirit to show in performance, that moment becomes something special—a moment when
the balance of all energies are at one. Then the singer is being sung.
Every practice, preparation for lessons, or performance, benefits from
taking a short moment to clear all the mind-talk, create a space for
openness to learning, and an attitude of gratitude for those gifts and
talents that are being encouraged and developed. When singers are too
busy criticizing their voices, they lose the ability to be grateful and de-
stroy the magic of the moment.

f) Physical aspects

The physical system includes all the physical and mechanical aspects
of the singer from the skeleton, muscles, nerves, organs, the brain,
to all the microscopic and macroscopic elements of the human body.
The vocal mechanism is more than the sum of its parts. This system
is energized and coordinated by all the other aspects of the energy
field.

Included in the physical system are: balance and whole body movement created by muscle actions, basic life rhythms such as breath
and heart beat, and movement at cellular, atomic and quantum levels.
When a singer only focuses on technique, the performance is often
stiff and boring, and the natural energies and rhythms of the body
are inhibited. Physical freedom is created by paying attention to the
collaboration of the six areas of the energy field discussed above.
Appropriate physical activity is important, but it is much more potent when the singer is in touch with natural reflexes, rhythms and
vibrations, all the invisible aspects of energy, and maintains a central
core of stillness.

Singers as masters of their own energy fields

It is easy to fall into the trap of thinking and feeling that the voice is simply part of the head and neck, and perhaps the chest. Ideal singing comes from being at one with the self, the surroundings, the music, and the spirit, coupled with a dynamic balance of the components of the vocal mechanism. How can singers accomplish this state of performance?

a) Take responsibility for learning

This involves looking carefully for a teacher that suits the needs and goals of the singer. It does not work to study with a well-known teacher if you are not compatible. A positive atmosphere for learning is critical for reaching optimum learning conditions.

Studying, practice and careful preparation are strictly the singer's responsibility—not the teacher's. Find ways to monitor learning. The most effective tool is the video. Singers who do not want to see themselves are at risk of fooling themselves and not communicating with the audience.

b) Take responsibility for thoughts and language

The energy field reacts strongly to the language used—in thought, written form, and in verbal expression. (More about this in Chapter 3).
Both singer and teacher will profit immensely when they take responsibility for their thinking and use of language in the studio, practice, and performance.

c) Pay mindful attention to each practice and lesson

Every practice session, and every lesson needs to have proper mental preparation. Preparation for teaching or singing includes creating an atmosphere or energy field that is supportive of a positive relationship between teacher and pupil or simply a good energy for accomplishing short-term goals. This can take the form of a short meditation, a moment to focus on each piece of music, thirty seconds of stillness before beginning.

d) Treat all colleagues, peers and teachers with respect

Have positive thoughts and actions towards, colleagues, peers, directors, and teachers. In the heat of a competitive environment, always stay centered within your own energy field. Do not waste emotions by getting involved even when they do not do the same for you. Negative emotional attachments can play havoc with your energy field and performance. Feeling sympathy is not the same as becoming emotionally attached.

e) Be centered and aware

Awareness will give you the ability to respond with clarity, spontaneity, and intuition—all needed for optimum learning and performance. Mind chatter, undue focus only on one thing, unnecessary emotional involvement, and repeated thought patterns are the demise of awareness.

There are many more aspects relating to the above five points to be discussed in Chapter 3. Times have changed so much that we can no longer afford to adhere to outdated pedagogical models for singing.

Vocal pedagogy in the 21ˢᵗ Century 3

As we enter the 21ˢᵗ Century, interest in the voice and singing is at an all time high. We are seeing rapid expansion of knowledge, new approaches to learning in all fields, various media and the Internet offer exposure to global vocal practices, and new avenues for vocal performance present themselves regularly. There are infinite numbers of possibilities available to us for teaching and learning. Information and the tools to make the teaching of singing far more efficient and exciting are readily available. Change is no longer an option; it is a necessity.

The combination of students who are more aware and the evolving vocal tastes of the general public are demanding change. The various reality shows about singing and the freedom for anyone to perform in public, on UTube or karaoke, are exposing the world to singing at its best and worst. Methods taught by the educated and uneducated are springing up for each style of singing creating an interesting dilemma. There are teachers who are still using methods that belong to the 19ᵗʰ century, some who have become ultra scientific and offer various ways of analyzing technique, either by system or machine, classical teachers who fear contemporary commercial music, and stylists in many popular genres who are trying to teach vocal technique when they have very little understanding of it. What is needed today to bring a more consistent quality to teaching and singing?

One option, suggested in the Introduction is: *Core Singing,* which uses the knowledge and understanding of all the aspects of the energy field to develop the student. To do this, change is needed in the way singing is approached and teachers are developed. It is possible to work first with the whole spectrum of energy in a variety of ways first to enable the joy and freedom of singing with the choice of style coming later. Current teaching of voice tends to be highly specialized. What is needed are some multi-faceted, generalist singing teachers who can give developing artists a core foundation of healthy vocal practice, expression, imagination and vocal options. The singer would then be free to choose a preferred style and move on to a specialist teacher.

In the discussion that follows we will look at some of the generic aspects of what is needed today by teachers and students. Topics include: working with the whole student, co-responsibility in learning, the issue of trust and the voice, the relationship of the language of teaching and the energy field, the role of self-development in teaching and learning, and the responsibilities of teachers and students.

Working with the *Whole* student

Everyone sings, or makes singing sounds; some of these people want to simply be better and others wish to make it their profession. Understanding this will help teachers enjoy the person who wants to sing, rather than the singer who is also a person. To be able to sing is a life-long wish of many who have been told they are not good enough. Any student who walks in a teacher's door is a gift to that teacher and deserves to be treated as such. The gratitude for the gift results in both teacher and singer working together to support the art and pleasure of singing rather than personal ego. When the teacher is grateful, it makes it possible for the singer also to look with gratitude on the lessons received. The student who has learned in this atmosphere will be a balanced performer because the lessons will be unforgettable. If the student goes on to become a professional singer that is at the same time co-incidental and a bonus.

Right – left brain balance in teaching and learning

What makes lessons interesting and unforgettable? The first requirement is balance of information, imagination and experience. Information goes into the analytical left-brain area described earlier as the "peanut", and experiences are processed in the right intuitive, creative brain. For example: the repetitive rote learning of the words to a song would involve only the left-brain, and the student might have difficulty remembering them. By learning text using visualization, movement, color, and other techniques, the right brain would also be engaged. The combination of both would imprint the text and music throughout the body and there would be less likelihood of memory slips. Many other areas of the brain are included when there is movement, color, imagination and so on. Langer (1997) states: *"Most often when we have learned something mindfully, we needn't worry about remembering it. The information is likely to be there when we need it"*.

Singers, other artists, and skilled athletes are more balanced than most because the mastery of their professions demands use of both sides of the brain. However even they are subjected to the academic and left-brain requirement of intellectual *proof.* Teachers have a difficult time separating what they have been taught for academic qualification and what they relay to students. Information overload is the best way to create bored students. It takes a clever teacher to be able to create practical learning experiences out of academic material.

Singing tends to encourage a balanced approach to learning because the left, language, brain, and the right, musical, brain both are needed for performance. Schools, colleges, and other institutions of learning are beginning to realize that new ways of training are needed to encourage the young to respond to information with curiosity and enthusiasm. The computer has changed everything about our lives, and that includes learning. Our education models have become more and more left-brain information oriented. The result is students (and this includes singers) who are walking encyclopedias of information without sufficient experience for that information to become knowledge.

Teaching that has a preponderance of information and little experience leaves the student with too little kinesthetic experience and in confusion as to what to do. Information based teaching often is full of right's, wrong's, and dogma which can lead to a rigid approach. Without adequate experience, students store the information in the left-brain, and believe it is the only way. Later when they are asked to perform differently, it is confusing, lowers their confidence, and they believe that they do not know how to respond.

"It's strange what we assume about learning. How often we pretend someone must force it upon us, and that we in turn must force it upon others. We get all tangled up in concepts and instructions. Can you remember when you first learned to ride a bicycle? Did anyone really help by trying to explain it to you?" Ristad (1982)

Learning to ride a bicycle involves doing it until you get the *feel* of it. Then one cannot remember when it wasn't possible to ride it. What happened between not knowing and knowing how to ride is similar to singing. It is a matter of sensory-motor understanding and almost any singer knows when he or she has it because it feels wonderful. There is then no question of trusting because each time riders/singers *get on the bicycle* they know it will be easy.

When singers are taught with a sense of "let's see what would happen if we did it this way", they are presented with choices in how to proceed. They can feel free to experiment on their own without guilt or a rigid protocol—even to "fall off the bicycle". This can create a temporary sense of instability. However as Langer (1997) says: *"For some, such uncertainty represents an absence of personal control. From a mindful perspective, however, uncertainty creates the freedom to discover meaning. If there are meaningful choices, there is uncertainty. If there is no choice, there is no uncertainty and no opportunity for control. The theory of mindfulness insists that uncertainty and the experience of personal control are inseparable more."*

Co-responsibility in learning and the establishment of trust

The studio presents an intimate situation in which two people, pupil and teacher, are there to create an artistic form of communication together. The achievement of this goal is equally important to both participants and a good relationship reflects the joint adventure.

From the beginning it is important to establish a clear understanding of the responsibilities of both teacher and student, as it is the first step toward maintaining personal power. Too often there is a situation where students give away their personal power to the teacher—and in some cases the teacher happily takes it. Singers will develop much more quickly when there are clear statements of what the teacher expects, and when the teacher finds out what the student expects. By establishing clear goals—even if the goals change later--students will be able to make informed choices in the way they learn, practice and relate to that teacher.

Ask the students what kind of sounds they would like to have? How might they describe their ideal voice? Taking the time to define a 'sound goal' is very useful and gets pupils thinking about their own unique voice- what qualities they want, how they want to be perceived as a person, by the audience, and so on. By establishing these goals, it gives students characteristics and values to monitor for themselves—especially when they are looking at a video of a lesson or performance.

The student has to learn to trust himself as well as the teacher. There is an intuitive 'knowing' in everyone and this is an important inner voice. *"How often we are robbed of our ecstasy by trusting implicitly in external authority and negating our internal wisdom ... We yield our wills and our imagination to experts, both visible and invisible, and pretend that only the experts have god-given powers of perception. We forget the legitimacy of our own knowing"* (Ristad, 1982).

The singer who has always depended on the teacher to determine the worth of a sound rarely will have complete confidence in performance. Performance anxiety and fear are created when there is a lack of trust about the act of singing. It is up to the teacher and student to find ways to develop an innate trust of the voice, to enjoy each sound without harsh judgment, to experience the pleasure of singing as a part of everyday life, and to carry that spirit into performance.

Use of language that enriches teaching and learning

The power of language is undeniable. The words we verbalize or think have a direct influence on the energy field of everyone around us. Therefore the teacher is responsible for not only what she says to the student, but also what she *thinks* when that student is in her presence. The language, attitudes, and thoughts of the teacher (and family) can contribute to/or inhibit the qualities of spontaneity, creativity and intuition.

The history of the teaching of singing has been fraught with a language pattern of negative criticism and the use of words such as: right-wrong, should-ought, control-hold, try, if and but. These words tend to create tension because the student does want to "get it right"; therefore creating stress and effort in the act of pleasing the teacher. More importantly this kind of vocabulary builds an "out of control" self-critic inside the person. While every artist needs an analytical and critical faculty, it is not possible to criticize oneself and sing at the same time without sacrificing spontaneity, creativity and intuition. Anything the singer is thinking other than the message will draw his or her own and the audience's attention away from the music. Certainly in the beginning, every pupil needs to be allowed to explore singing in a joyful, supportive manner. While notes, rhythms and musical indications are important, it is much more freeing to begin with simple improvisation where correctness is not so critical. Making sound that is not restricted by musical or vocal constraints (other than vocal health) promotes confidence. Later the need to be accurate can be addressed in ways that are positive and exciting. However, first let the singer sing for the love of it. This will allow an open, honest communication to be established between teacher and pupil and give the student real motivation to improve. In this environment imagination, humor, fun, and hard work will flourish.

The comfort of the student in a learning situation goes a long way toward the elimination of self-sabotage on the part of the singer. The inner and outer language of the teacher helps establish an example of mental and verbal discipline that the singer will follow. For example, when a teacher tells a student a song is hard, the student will find it more than a challenge to learn. When the singer thinks a certain high note always will be difficult, it will be. It becomes a self-fulfilling prophecy. What we think and say becomes reality. It is up to the teacher and student to create both a viable and enjoyable reality with a positive and encouraging use of language.

Self-development as the core of teaching and learning

Singing is a powerful tool for self-realization and for nourishment of others. Developing it is a shared responsibility. Curiosity about life and learning is a wonderful asset for the teacher. It creates the energy necessary to pursue information, new experiences, and the enthusiasm of sharing with colleagues and students. When there is a commitment to curiosity, teaching and learning become magical. One discovery leads to another and another and another—the love of learning never stops.

A teacher who spends time on her own self-development as an important and integral part of her work—rather than something "I will do when I have the time" has much more to offer students. Academic requirements and/or performance experience are only the beginning of the development of a teacher of singing or a singer. It is every voice professional's responsibility to be educated as fully as possible, and not to depend on current or long established curricula to do it all. The teaching of singing is not just a skill for those who have sung professionally; neither can the academic environment present the prospective teacher with all that is needed. It is simply not enough. The 21st century is an era when self-development and new awareness of infinite possibilities are guiding many on personal journeys of inner and outer discovery. Every discovery is useful in teaching and learning.

As singing involves every aspect of a person, ranging from the physical to the spiritual, performers and voice professionals owe it to themselves to develop every part of themselves over time. Each new aspect enriches the person in visible and invisible ways. There are an infinite variety of personal development tools available today: Alexander technique, fitness classes, sport, applied kinesiology, many useful psychological techniques such as NLP, meditation, Qigong, and Tai chi, Yoga, and much more.

Self-development presents the voice professional with the opportunity to become a whole person who is centered, open, aware, emotionally mature, non-judgmental, a good communicator, and to teach and/or perform from a place of service, gratitude and love. This is a direct challenge to voice professionals and developing singers to take responsibility for their own personal growth and know that ultimately what is known has to come from the inside.

The responsibility of the teacher

Most people who enjoy teaching do so because they loved being a student and they want to help others enjoy it too. Singing teachers have an additional asset; they have a passion for their art. Most consider it a gift to be associated with singing and music on a daily basis. The teacher of singing has certain obligations to this gift by continuing to learn, pursuing personal development, being diligent about the atmosphere in the studio or clinic, and being professional in approach. These responsibilities are outlined further below.

a) Continue to be a lifelong student

The well-balanced teacher of singing approaches vocal education in a manner that couples curiosity and wonder with knowledge of artistry, function, physical balance, excellent communication skills, emotional detachment to any outcomes, and the ability to honor and value each student. This multi-faceted approach to singing will enable teachers and students to creatively develop their artistry.

When teaching techniques are derived from comprehension of fundamental principles and a multi-faceted approach, rather than some process learned by rote that becomes more distorted as it moves through succeeding generations of teachers and singers, creative and enjoyable lessons can be learned. Since each student has individual vocal needs, that student cannot be taught to sing properly unless these needs are singled out and dealt with intelligently.

The balance that comes from a multi-layered or core singing approach is necessary for the stability and the encouragement of naturalness in the singer. With so much information coming from all directions, it is easy to become confused or emphasize only one facet. Dedicated study and integration will ensure that vocal function, personal development, and artistry are part of the whole and do not need to be separated.

It is the teacher's responsibility to learn the many facets of the human voice so that his perception of the personality, voice and learning style of the pupil is informed enough to provide that student with efficient and significant coaching.

Obvious problems of posture, breathing, attack, resonance and articulation can be resolved by a teacher with a basic understanding of how these matters are determined physiologically. Many singer's problems can be observed visually in their posture, breathing patterns, and tensions in the arms, chest, neck and face. Since these problems are *physical* and *sensory*, it is virtually impossible to change them with verbal instructions only. The student has to sense the difference in order to change. The teacher needs to understand that it is not always possible to verbalize what is physical or kinesthetic because it is an experience.

The teacher who is well versed in physiological and psychological matters will be severely limited unless there is also a sympathetic understanding of artistry. In the final analysis, it is a performer's artistry and magnetism that provide the essential elements needed for communication. Therefore, it is important for a teacher to have performed in public (that is not to say he must have been famous, only that he has performed publicly in a variety of situations and can understand and analyze those elements of artistry necessary to fine singing). It is equally important to keep his ear educated by continually attending performances by fine artists in a variety of genres, and to familiarize himself with the literature of the voice and of other performing arts. Today a professional singer is expected to be versatile and so must the teacher.

b) Learn to coach the mental aspects of performance

Every good athlete has a coach or special trainer to teach him how to focus on his goals and perform under pressure. When it works well, they call it being in the zone—that state of awareness where the performance is seemingly automatic and without thought. At the moment, student singers sometimes get there by accident and professionals get there from experience. Neither of them knows how to recreate the sensation. This is something the arts need to borrow from sport education because it is part of optimum performance in any field. There are many methods and therapies such as visualization, meditation, NLP, specialist psychologists and many others that teach mental preparation. Mental preparation is an important aspect of learning and performing. The wise teacher will use these techniques in the lesson and teach the student to use them in every practice session.

c) Create a positive studio atmosphere for learning and performing by having a physical, mental, emotional and spiritual safe haven for every student

The teacher who has an aware, open, non-judgmental attitude provides an empathetic and congenial studio atmosphere where optimum learning is fostered. A relationship based on spirit, art and humanity rather than self-importance, ego and vanity will supply the student with a superb model.

The voice professional must deal often with a sensitive human instrument and be aware of potential self-consciousness of the student in a vulnerable situation. It is important to allow trial and error and accept the temporary consequences. Affording the singer a safe haven to experiment, rather than to have to get it right, encourages confidence. It is such positive support and encouragement that reinforces proper technique and artistry. Bullying and threats do not belong in the teaching or performance environments. Ideally each lesson will provide at least one positive accomplishment, either technical or musical, that can be taken away from the studio and retained. This is how ideas are remembered and practiced long after the lesson is finished.

d) Be grateful for each student

It is easy to forget to be grateful and necessary to make a practice of it (Byrne, 2006). There is something to be learned from everyone. When it is a privilege to teach a student, the student will sense it and respond with trust, confidence, a sense of wellbeing and a heightened ability to produce his best effort. Often, teachers temporarily forget to be grateful because they become lost in the day-to-day pattern of work, making a living, dealing with family, performing, and a myriad of other things.

Take responsibility to dedicate each day and each lesson with a moment of silence or visualization about what you want from that day. Thirty seconds at the beginning of each lesson will set the scene for centered teaching and learning. Students likely will need a moment to settle before a lesson, and this offers a meaningful opportunity.

e) Be professional about the business of singing

Performing artists and those who teach them are not always known for their business acumen. However, it is time that such acumen became a part of every voice professional's tool kit. Good marketing, studio mission statements, what the student will get, what is expected of the student, and clear policies about pricing and learning, all help the prospective student to know whether to work with a teacher. This is just the beginning. Treat your students as if they were valued business clients and provide an uncluttered studio for them. Dress as if they were special as well.

Provide a clearly written brochure or website providing information about the following:

- The mission of your teaching (or therapeutic practice)
- Whether you specialize in a specific style or you prefer working with core singing.
- Are you willing to offer consultations, trial lessons and short-term packages?
- What you offer: private sessions, group lessons, repertoire class, etc.
- Are there age preferences?
- The "rules" of your studio regarding lessons, arriving late, missed lessons, and payments.
- Include a short paragraph about your background

Students (and their parents, when appropriate) are entitled to know what is expected when they study with a teacher. This can be aided by creating a simple contract between teacher and student—that can be broken when it is not being met on either side. Those who teach in university may be somewhat limited in this regard, however, in addition to the applied lesson syllabi, other expectations can be discussed and agreed at the beginning of each term.

Be clear about your requirements and be honest when they are not working. It is not the teacher or the student's fault; it is simply not a good match. Treat it as a business rather than something that is based on blame or guilt. Allow consultation lessons with no strings attached. Make it easy by offering a contract for a series or package of five or ten lessons. This will give both teacher and student a fair amount of time to make an informed decision as to whether to continue.

Consult with others in the field for advice and use their services when it is appropriate. It is common practice in business and sport. It was reported that a team of four sports-science experts accompanied the American swimmers at the 2008 Beijing Olympics. Each race was videotaped. Immediately after a race, each swimmer had an ear pricked to test for lactic-acid levels (relates to muscle soreness). After a warm-down swim, video analysis was made available to monitor stroke counts, distance per stroke, split times, and the biomechanics of take-offs and turns.

Singers do not need to have such a large team or analyze so much detail, however a video review of lessons and performances would be invaluable. Video feedback now is considered a part of sports training whether it is team or individual. Performers profit greatly from video feedback because they get used to seeing themselves as they are, not as they *think* they are. Teachers very rarely have to justify corrections when the student has seen and heard the change on video.

The responsibility of the student

The responsibility for each lesson and learning lies equally in the hands of the student. The ideal student comes equipped with curiosity to explore new ideas and ways of singing, the ability to listen, the courage to use his imagination and take creative risks, mindful practice habits, and dedication to his art.

The main areas of co-responsibility for the singer are outlined below.

a) Objectivity

It is important that both the student and the teacher view singing with objectivity rather than something personal. For example, if an instrumentalist has a dent on his flute, he does not usually take it personally, but takes it to someone who can correct it. Yes, the flute does not live inside that person like the voice, but the voice can be treated as an instrument in the same way. Corrections suggested by the teacher are not directed at the person but towards the improvement of the voice. The student must learn to separate him/herself as an individual from the voice as an instrument, so that objective learning rather than subjective inhibitions will take place.

When the voice is perceived one way by the singer, and another by the instructor a coaching problem is created. Students have to be nonjudgmental and take the responsibility for finding ways to objectively see and hear what differences the corrections make.

This is especially necessary for singers who have preconceived ideas regarding their sound (such as very heavy and full, or very light) when their concept differs from the teacher's. For example, the lyric soprano who pushes her voice to sound heavy in order to sing like a dramatic soprano because she thinks that is *her* sound, or the baritone who is really a tenor who is misguided or led into believing that his sound is bigger and deeper than that which the physiological structure of his instrument would indicate.

The ability to be objective frees the student from unwanted emotional interference with learning and correction. Come to the lesson with a clean computer screen ready for new information. Later it will be possible to analyze the information and decide whether to delete or save.

b) Extra-curricula development complementary to singing

Find a way to learn skills that are complementary to singing such as dance and movement, piano, acting, languages, Qigong, Tai chi, Alexander technique and many others. Some advanced schools and universities are including some of these activities in their curricula. Where they are not, singers need to find their own way to pursue these activities.

c) Elimination of mind chatter and excessive self-criticism

As discussed in Chapter 2, the language you think and verbally express has a powerful effect on the energy field and whether or not goals are achieved. Mind chatter while singing is the equivalent of trying to perform in competition with a radio. It stifles awareness and spontaneity. Perceptions of music being difficult, notes being hard to reach, fear of making a mistake will all perpetuate the problem. Using visualization, and mental focus can eliminate self-fulfilling prophecies. Know and state what is wanted; not that which is unwanted. Learn to talk to yourself differently.

Being a good student means having the courage to leap into the unknown. *"It takes an act of will to become vulnerable enough to explore scary, unknown territory in our minds and bodies ... It takes will power and courage to suffer the turmoil of change. As long as we return to our old habits/formulas we will not take the step into unfamiliar territory."* *(Ristad, 1982)*

Exploring the unknown means leaving the "self-critic" on the doorstep when one walks into the teaching studio. The analysis can be left to the teacher and any self-analysis allowed to wait until the lesson is finished. A noisy internal dialogue prohibits hearing and spontaneity, severely limits the imagination and the ability to respond freely and therefore creates singing perceived as rigid and fixed. An open mind with no pre-conceived ideas is a primary requisite for learning to sing. An aspiring artist must enter the studio with a sense of personal freedom that is tied to a serious commitment to his art.

d) Meaningful practice and rehearsal

Good results can be obtained from every practice session, whether it lasts for five minutes or more than an hour. The key to this is to know what you want to achieve during each session. Take a moment to sit quietly and visualize the objectives before beginning the session or each song.

e) Find ways to monitor progress

Do not be afraid to look at yourself. It is the only way you will know whether you are fulfilling your own objectives in singing and performance. It can be a rude shock when someone ridicules or does not like what you produced. Singers who perform in genres outside the classical arena seem to be comfortable in looking at themselves. However, classical singers are far behind in this aspect of their learning. Every student needs a way to video lessons and important rehearsals and to view them objectively. This is a key area where the singer can take personal responsibility for monitoring the effectiveness of his study and performance.

f) Have the courage to take performance risks

Good singers and performers do not "play it safe and try to get it right". They participate fully in creating and being part of a meaningful performance experience. Very rarely does a developing singer go too far. When viewed as an experiment, every correction or new option that presents itself will be exciting. Viewed objectively, if it works, it can be used; if not, it can be forgot. *"A lot of singers think all they have to do is exercise their tonsils to get ahead. They refuse to look for new ideas and new outlets, so they fall by the wayside... I'm going to try to find out the new ideas before the others do."* Ella Fitzgerald. When spirit, art, and humanity, are the basis for learning, rather than self-importance, ego and vanity, singers will learn all they need to know and will be able to take such risks.

g) Be grateful for your talent

When a singer is grateful for her voice, it becomes easy to sing. Self- and voice bashing is not an option if a singer wants to progress. The mental and psychological result of such personal bashing is a recipe for discouragement and a long, slow road to progress. As Ella Fitzgerald has said: *"I know I'm no glamour girl, and it's not easy for me to get up in front of a crowd of people. It used to bother me a lot, but now I've got it figured out that God gave me this talent to use, so I just stand there and sing."*

The future of vocal pedagogy

For the past thirty years there has been a movement towards greater scientific accuracy by the teachers of singing and voice, particularly those in colleges and universities. In fact, so much, that in some instances the teaching of voice has become clinical and more like voice therapy than singing. Now, due to the increased awareness about the function of the body/mind/energy field in dance and sport and the use of adjunct techniques like Alexander lessons, BodyMapping™, BrainGym™, body work, martial arts, and energy field healing, the teaching of singing is expanding in many directions. In the future we will see an exciting combination of the arts, sciences, sport, psychology, and healing used in teaching. This cannot help but broaden our knowledge and perceptions resulting in a more efficient way to teach and to perform.

What are some of the changes needed to make this shift towards a more efficient teaching and learning of the art of singing?

- A new look at the balance of the relationship of the art of singing and science
- The establishment of generalist teachers that teach core singing
- Active partnership with the student
- The inclusion of helpful performance techniques borrowed from the Eastern practices such as Qigong, tai chi, martial arts, and sport
- Research in the above areas to stimulate creative new investigations into performance
- More consultations among voice professionals
- Balanced singers who perform with the mental focus of skilled athletes

As the changes above manifest, singers will have a renewed sense and balance of their personal space and energy field, will have a true presence—being completely in the now—responsive to the message, the music and the audience.

The singer of the 21st Century will be a multi-dimensional singer whose energy field, and therefore her voice, will fill and permeate space and with the capacity to thrill, excite, and heal those who have come to listen and take part.

"When a human being brings forth a tone or a sound, his whole organism is actually involved, and what takes place in the song ... is only the final culmination of what goes on within the entire human being."
Steiner (1983)

What every singer needs to know: Co-ordination, spontaneity and artistry 4

While each singer is responsible for the awareness, the feeling and sense of performance, much can be learned from the experiences of some of the greats. Singers who perform in public on a regular basis, get a feel for performance in a way that few others can. Some of their descriptions are quoted in the paragraphs of this chapter. Great athletes experience something similar when they have to give of their best in front of thousands of people all the time. They have something to offer performing artists as well. For anyone aspiring to sing, it is helpful to learn about the experiences of famous performers in a variety of fields.

The public is constantly exposed to many types and varieties of vocal music through recordings, theater, radio and television and they expect quality performance. The public can at the same time be adoring and supportive, and fickle and demanding. *"The audience is the best judge of anything. They cannot be lied to. Truth brings them closer. A moment that lags – they're gonna cough"*. (Barbara Streisand) A singer must be versatile enough to satisfy public demand and to cope with the harsh reality of insufficient work to support artists in only one type of performance, such as recitals or cabaret. Until established, young singers have to be prepared to do anything that comes their way. Those who cannot see the value of versatility often excuse their lack of success by blaming everyone else for their failures. In 1924, Greene said: *"It seems inconceivable that a thing of great beauty, a great gift like a voice, should count for nothing in the world of music, and the singer in his disappointment attributes his failure to the shortcomings of his manager, the opportunities of his rivals, the personal prejudices of his critics or the restlessness of the gods – to anything but the true cause. The explanation is simple enough – he has not learned his business."*
Today the business of music is more complex than ever. Singers have numbers of possible avenues for development: from musical theater, cruise ships, cabaret, singer/songwriter, radio, television, recitals, oratorios and opera to Internet performance. The more versatile they are,

the more options there will be, and the better the chances of financial survival. *"What makes my approach special is that I do different things. I do jazz, blues, country music and so forth. I do them all, like a good utility man"* (Ray Charles).

The "business" of singing, apart from healthy vocal production, involves musicianship, style, knowledge of dialects and languages, personal development and excellent communication skills. For singing in most styles and classical formats such as opera and giving recitals, competence in skills such as languages, dancing, acting, mime and the ability to play an instrument are invaluable. The more skills the singer possesses the better chance of a performing career.

The underlying physiological principles of vocal technique are important and helpful for singer to understand and to apply them intelligently to his or her own needs. While this will increase the singer's chances for a purer, more efficient voice, the making of an artist requires much more. To elevate technique into an art there must be co-ordination that allows freedom in performance, spontaneity that springs from confidence and knowledge, and personal magnetism to attract the listeners.

Co-ordination

The essence of vocal technique has been realised when all of the physiological, mental, and emotional factors work harmoniously to produce the desired tone in a spontaneous and dynamic manner. This co-ordination and skill are achieved with proper direction, hard work, and patient, disciplined practice, In writing about his famous pupil Kathleen Ferrier, Henderson said: *"Every art has its own technique and Kathleen had to learn the craft before the artist in her rose to conceal the hard work of the studio"* (Cardus, 1954).

Some prima donnas like Sills, Farrell and Horne, and more recently singers like Flemming, Terfel, and Dessay, were performing at very young ages and they had to work diligently. The same is true for singers of contemporary commercial music like Celine Dion who commented: *"There has been nothing but discipline, discipline, discipline all my life."* There is no easy road to unfailingly good vocal technique. Legouvé (in Gattey, 1979) described Malibran's struggle with vocal technique: *"Every now and then she stopped short to scold her own voice saying, 'Obey me'. The struggle was therefore a necessity and had become a habit which, added to her invincible tenacity and her love for doing that which seemed impossible, invested her talent with much more powerful and original character ..."*

Malibran worked ceaselessly, and Gattey (1979) pointed out that in so doing she proved the corollary of the saying, "A prima donna who rests, rusts", however, inadequate rest is also harmful. Malibran's exhausting schedule of practice from 9am–10am, theatre rehearsal from 10am–1pm, concerts from 2pm–4pm, opera from 7pm–10pm, followed by late night concerts probably contributed to her untimely death at the age of 29.

In the past, singers could rely on performance being preceded by scores of rehearsals. In this fast-moving jet age, unless a new work is being presented, the number of rehearsals can be as few as three. A singer without a firmly established technique has little chance of developing it under these circumstances. Most opera singers do not perform regularly until they are in their late twenties or thirties; by that time they have learned the value and method of proper practice. On the other hand many performers of popular music are evanescent because they begin at an early age, some are poorly trained; they tend to work in emotionally overcharged atmospheres for long hours and they may "burn out" before they develop their full potential.

Long hours of practice risk endangering the voice because of the limitations of the muscles involved and the expenditure of energy required. The actual singing time of practice may be limited to avoid over tiring the voice. On the other hand there is no limitation of time for the 'academic' aspect of practice which includes learning the rhythm, meaning, and pronunciation of the text, memorising the text and music, and understanding the conceptual and emotional content of the song.

Spontaneity

Over and above co-ordinated technique, a spontaneous natural performance requires musicianship, interpretation, movement and acting. Musicianship involves the ability to read music, play an instrument, and sight-sing. Under ideal circumstances these skills will have been learned and established before vocal study begins. It is a waste of time for a singing teacher to have to teach musicianship rather than the techniques and artistry of singing. The study of piano (or other instruments) imbues the performer with a sense of rhythm, phrasing and style, and makes it easier for him to learn vocal music and collaborate with accompanists. Malibran, Melba, Ferrier, and many pop artists like Josh Groban, Billy Joel and Elton John have played so well that they have been able to accompany themselves and keep their vocal learning time at a minimum. It was easy for them to learn notes and rhythms.

The singer who can sight-sing well has the potential for reproducing the score in his head and practising it without uttering a sound. Except for establishing a certain pitch, he rarely needs to use the piano, and his ability to pick up a new work and sing it with some confidence eliminates much of the physical tension associated with learning. Daily practice of sight-singing a new song maintains the skill. Session singers get paid a lot of money for their sight-singing ability in the recording studio.

According to Greene (1924) the interpreter of music must have acquired and perfected technique, the gift of magnetism, an inborn or assimilated sense of atmosphere and a command of tone-colour. Interpretation is effective when all the elements of a song are treated interdependently. The serious singer cannot function properly without studying the language, history and style of every piece in his repertoire. It is not enough to know the general intent or meaning of a song: every phrase and sentence must be understood.

For the classical singer, this requires a working knowledge of English, Italian, French and German including diction and basic grammar – anything less is a waste of time. Balk (1985) in his book *The Complete Singer-Actor* wrote: *"The student may know that the aria is about the loss of love, or some such gloss of overall meaning, but that vital second-to-second, word-to-word understanding essential to communication, to drama, and to music is absent a great share of the time. We encourage one of the worst mental habits the young singer-actor can acquire by our tolerance of un-integrated, unincorporated work in a foreign language… It is important to note, however, that opera training demands not only a specific knowledge, word by word and phrase by phrase, of what is happening before, behind, and around the words and how they can be colored and inflected to convey all their meanings."*

Singing a song without understanding every word is comparable to reciting a shopping list. The better the singer knows the language, the more efficient is the learning of the song. Finally, the singer who learns these four languages well can more easily add repertoire in less frequently used languages like Spanish, Russian and Czech. Latin is essential for liturgical and oratorio singers.

Knowledge of grammar is important for correct phrasing. Singers who ignore the punctuation and grammar of the text, will take breaths in the middle of a prepositional phrase, between subject and predicate, or worse still, will sing through periods (full stops) and important commas just to demonstrate how much breath they have. Since communication is the ultimate aim of singing, the performer must be as cognisant of the rhythm inherent in the language and text as he is of the rhythm of the music. His art is not a demonstration of breathing technique.

A background in the history of music is valuable; it provides knowledge of the stylistic characteristics of the period and composers. Singers are expected to give valid stylistic performances. In performance it is important to know which composers allowed improvised coloratura and what they demanded in ornamentation and rubato. A study of the composer, his music and times will reveal this information and will provide insight into texts that often hold little meaning for contemporary singers. Knowledge of history and style will contribute much to the relevance and vitality of a performance, yet never impose fussy detail or self-conscious effects which both cheapen performance and interfere with communication of the music to the audience.

Acting ability lends the spontaneity to a singer's performance that ultimately leads to better interpretation. Even when the singer does not use large gestures and staging during a recital, the ability to imagine the action enhances the interpretation. Hubert Kockritz demonstrated the value of such imagination in a number of workshops held for the National Association of Teachers of Singing in the United States. He asked a young singer to perform a song first in the recital position in the crook of the piano. Then he reset the song with some stage properties, movement and gestures and coached the performer until it was sung to his satisfaction. The singer was then asked to return to the original position to sing without any of the adjustments. The difference between the first and last performance was a dramatic indication of the value of a mental picture in improving interpretation, vocal technique and communication of the song to the audience. The imagination is one of the most neglected tools of singing—in every style.

Dramatic training involves the study of body language, movement, and the emotional and psychological aspects of the text. The keen performer is willing to do anything that is asked of him on stage and do it convincingly. It is his responsibility.

Long before serious vocal training begins, a potential singer would do well to enroll in movement and dance classes where he can cultivate a sense of rhythm and of dynamic movement. (Natalie Dessay began as a ballet dancer) The absence of appropriate movement can ruin a concert or operatic performance with the singer's entrance even before a note is sung. In her delightful book, In My Own Key, Söderström (1979) speaks forcefully about the importance of using the body properly.

"Learn to use your body ... hands, feet, large gestures ... and do them in front of a mirror. I think there is a great pity that there is not more teaching of 'body language' all over the world. When I see a performance by a singer with a fantastic voice, but who cannot differentiate between a positive and negative gesture, then that gesture should defi-

nitely not be used. When I think of the thousands of hours artists spend polishing their voices, it seems to me almost criminal to let them appear in opera without knowing how to use body language on stage."

The current interest in movement and dance has been accompanied by an abundance of classes available during the day and at night. There are quality courses in conditioning, movement, modern dance, jazz and classical ballet, and yoga and tai chi. Before enrolling in a class, the student would be wise to ascertain that the teacher's credentials are sound. A voice capable of freedom is an extension of a body and mind with the same ability; and a song can be better communicated when the singer has the skill to add an appropriate look or a full-fledged gesture.

Balk (1985) attaches fundamental importance to the integration of many factors which include the whole individual as well as the performing actor and singer, the total environment of theater and audience, the music, the words and their interpretation. Meeting these exacting demands provides an exciting and fulfilling work of artistry.

In many young singers, technique and emotion are poorly co-ordinated, with physical and vocal tension often incorrectly substituted for emotion. Even a minor role requires specific characterisation. The artificiality of opera and the hyperactivity of contemporary commercial music are convincing only when the performers are genuine, natural and masters and mistresses of the dramatic and musical situation. This precludes interference from mental and physical tensions, and the adaptation of excessive or stylised posturing, all of which mar and detract from the real and intimate communication that exists between singers and audience.

There are three essential elements for credible performance: concentration, purpose and confidence. Concentration implies a total commitment of emotional, mental, and vocal resources where the words effect the sound and tone-colour, the drama is transmitted, and the character's movements and actions have purpose and intensity. When the singer's eyes wander, for example, so will an audience's attention, because the singer himself will have lost his bearings. Both purpose and concentration when added to a viable vocal technique and skilled performance will give the singer the confidence to sing well. As the singer develops and matures in his craft, each small victory he achieves will whittle away at any vestiges of inhibition or self-consciousness that remain.

With the mastery of technique, acting, and movement, more spontaneity is experienced. What remains is to exercise intuitive faculties and release that indefinable aspect of any performance-artistry.

Artistry

Throughout the literature on great singers who have had the courage to be creative and have dared to be free in their art, there are repeated references to certain characteristic traits shared by all: a great love of singing, dedication to work and emotional involvement in it. Almost all are or were strong individualists with magnetic personalities arousing empathy in the audience that defies definition.

a) Love of singing

"The only thing better than singing is more singing" (Ella Fitzgerald).
Facing a public, sometimes adoring or critical, takes a great presence and true love of art which are so well illustrated by three quotations from Söderström (1979):
"How can I describe the ecstasy you feel when every fibre in your body vibrates on the same wave length as the notes, when a high C-sharp suddenly sparkles in front of you as if a sun had appeared in the auditorium ..."
"My own sense of happiness seemed to be infectious, because the audience was 'struck' just as forcibly as I was myself ..."
"I stand on a platform to sing to and not for an audience. This has nothing to do with snobbery or attempts to educate people. It is an intense desire to be allowed to share the worlds of beauty from which I myself derive such endless stimulation."

b) Dedication to the work of singing

Long hours in preparation for comparatively brief moments on stage require rigorous self-discipline. The hours of rehearsal, travel, jet-lag, unfamiliar surroundings and inconsistent schedule require true dedication, as indicated by W. Ferrier (1955) in discussing her sister, Kathleen. She suggests that there can be no formal training for living the life of a singer. The experience demands constant attention, energy and thought.

c) Individuality

Personality traits of great singers have always ranged from rare and delightful humility to the supremely egotistical.

"Singing brings out in me what I can't normally bring out in every day life. It's an incredible feeling to be able to bare your soul to people you've never met in a way that can make them understand so clearly what you mean. That's what I love about singing...it becomes my truest form of communication" (Josh Groban).

Both Banti and Catalini were noted for their self-centered contempt for others. Banti conversed *mezzo voce* with the performers in the orchestra whenever she herself was not singing in a scene. Catalini thought nothing of violating the musical score in order to bolster her role. Her fee was so high that when concert managers complained that they could not afford to hire other good artists for the same production, her husband replied: *"Does it matter? In my view the best possible opera company consists of my wife and a few puppets"* (Gattey, 1979).

Malibran was known to have relaxed at home by leaping over chairs and tables. *"When I try to restrain my flow of spirits, I feel as if I should be suffocated"* (Gattey, 1979). Today's prima donnas cannot afford, and often, choose not to practice the foibles of their predecessors. Kathleen Ferrier was loved by all who worked with her – scene shifters, conductors and choirs. She was thoughtful, modest and part of a united company bent on giving a good performance: the music was predominant; the performers and their helpers, the instruments, and all were important to her. Beverley Sills was auditioned at least five or six times for the New York City Opera. She refused to be discouraged and was finally accepted. She had a distinguished career, and a special brightness and ability to articulate what performance means to a variety of people. Singers need a strong will and perseverance to survive not only the rigours of the art, but also the intense competition in the field; and when this is combined with the perspective of genuine and perceptive humility and gratitude there will be many helping hands.

d) Emotional involvement

Communication with an audience depends a great deal on the inspiration provided by the singer. *"If I am not feeling inspired, am not on good form, or am not sufficiently prepared"*, said Söderström (1979), *"then I can kill a piece of music before it has a chance to live"*. Berlioz said that an unimaginative singer is a "performer on the larynx" (in Gattey, 1979).

e) Personality and magnetism

The attraction of a singer to an audience is difficult to define, and critics refer as often to the personality and magnetism of singers as to any other features. Balk (1985) speaks of charisma as being the ability to project energy. Lind was described as a "thin, pale, plain-featured girl looking awkward and nervous" (Gattey, 1979). However, when she sang, her face and figure were transformed and illuminated "with the whole fire and dignity of her genius" (Legouvé discussing Lind in Gattey, 1979).

References like these abound in books about singers. Literature regarding any of the great singers constantly reminds the reader of his or her own special magnetism that goes beyond the voice, musicianship and interpretative powers.

f) Performance that transcends the ordinary

The elation of concert goers who have experienced a special moment of sublime artistry has often inspired them to try to put into words what they felt and heard.

"As for myself, I felt like a man in the car of a balloon at the moment they let go the ropes … darting into space like an arrow from a bow. It is the only way I can describe my feelings. Up till then music with me had been a gentle art, graceful and spirited. It now appeared to me as a most pathetic and purest vehicle for interpreting the deepest emotions. A new world had been revealed – the world of dramatic music" (Lagouvé on hearing Malibran, in Gattey, 1979).

"Suddenly the concert was transformed into divine worship; I don't know how to describe it. Time stood still and you feel it a favour to be allowed to be alive and experience such supernatural beauty" (Söderström, 1979 on hearing another's performance).

It is for moments like those described above that the singer spends long years of preparation. It is for his own satisfaction that he or she begins the training, the study, the remoulding of mind and body into a finely-tuned instrument. What remains then is for the singer through self-discipline to release the artist and become a dynamic performer.

On becoming a dynamic singer

Sound itself is dynamic and constantly changing, altering also in relation to the position and movement of performer and hearer. According to Winckel (1967): *"The intoned individual sound alone has such a dynamic life that after the lapse of one second both form and necessarily also timbre will have changed"*. He goes on to state how exact uniformity of amplitude and intensity of sound can be very unpleasant (for example, strictly periodic vibrato or trill are unbearable to the listener). Such exactness imposes a rigid law on a work of art from outside which makes creative power illusory or is prejudicial to its operation. Creativity must have discipline and yet it is killed by regimented uniformity. Music, when well-performed, has a way of overcoming this by being timeless and giving one a sense of being lifted out of oneself. The dynamic performer steps out of himself and allows this timelessness to pervade his being so that intuitive faculties take over and creativity flows from within and his making of music is a flowing, ever changing, spontaneous entity. This creativity and spontaneity does not preclude thorough grounding in aspects of technique, musicianship and the skills necessary for performance. As Govinda (1977) has so aptly stated1:

"Those who think that any conscious effort or aspiration is a violation of our spontaneous genius, and who look down upon any technique or method or the fruits of traditional experience as below their dignity, only deceive themselves and others. We can be spontaneous and fully conscious of the forms and forces of tradition.

We do not free ourselves from our past by trying to forget or ignore it, but only through mastering it in the light of higher, i.e. unprejudicial knowledge."

Dynamism comes from true mental receptivity and sensitivity. Being dynamic implies a body that moves gracefully; a technique that is ever-changing within the framework of vocal production and emotion; awareness of what one's senses are conveying from within and without; a sense of unconfined space and certain imperfections which add uniqueness to the performance.

A body, mind, and spirit that are free, are fluid in the ability to respond to the immediate environment and emotional situation of the moment. This defines the dynamic tension and release necessary to the creative artist. Such freedom allows the technique of singing to respond to living experience and direct perception. This ever-changing responsive mechanism then ensures clarity of voice, correct vocal attack and tone-colour, all of which respond to the moment-to-moment thoughts, emotions, and spirit of the singer.

The ideas and emotions are fed by the performer's heightened awareness and sensitivity to the information he is deriving from external and internal, visible and invisible sources. The numerous sensory receptors located in the ears, eyes, skin, joints, ligaments, muscles, tissues of the body constantly relay information to the brain and energy field. Such information is important because it is the key to the interplay of all the invisible and physical factors involved in performance.

Heightened creative sensitivity is gained only by the performer who has achieved a sense of inner quietude which allows the information to become apparent. This information is available to everyone, unfortunately many do not "hear" it because they are deafened by internal "noise". The causes of this noise are many but include excessive intellectualising and egocentricity. Whatever the cause, there are periods when it is essential for the singer to withdraw and achieve his own quiet and inner peace so that he is in touch with his own being in mind and body.

The singer who achieves this awareness of his own being gains a new and truer sense of perspective. Like the creative dancer he will appreciate the space in which he has to perform. This space is difficult to discuss because it is neither visible nor tangible – just as music is neither visible nor tangible. There are many aspects of space the performer may sense: his own personal, physical and psychic space; and those of time, sound and movement.

This so-called space is created and maintained by the performer's concentration and sensitivity to music, emotion, and his own intuition and creativity. When such an atmosphere is achieved then confidence, commitment, and communication with the audience become apparent. There is a magnetic empathy between performer and audience, as well as a feeling of nothing being absolute.

"In fact, Western music produces a kind of space-sensation which is remote from visible space as is that which is experienced in states of deep absorption. It is a space-experience which cannot be experienced in terms of three dimensions, because it belongs to a higher order ..." (Govinda, 1977).

A singer who experiences this profound perception of space feels no absolute measures of any aspect of performance – pitch, loudness, time or movement. He is at the same time lost, yet truly free – the most difficult achievement in all of performing. It is this letting go physically and emotionally and the willingness to be "lost" that determines finally just how dynamic the singer will become. Everyone wants something on which to anchor – technique, rhythm, time and ideas – yet by holding on one becomes static. *"Whatever we master, we need not cling to; we can always create it anew"* (Govinda, 1977). To lose oneself or to let go means that certain imperfections will occur – nothing will be the same. There is the oft repeated rule in singing that no two notes, phrases or words are to be sung exactly the same way because it introduces boredom and a certain static quality of performance. Differences will naturally occur because perfection is impossible. As a result the performance may not always meet the singer's own demands, instead it will take on special qualities indicative of that person. Winckel (1967) in describing sound mentions that there are often unintended components of sound, some of which deviate from pure harmony. These he calls a necessary "seasoning in the dish". This seasoning in singing may resemble technical and emotional imperfections to the artist yet it will often give special qualities to a performance.

The dynamic singer strives to perfect his art by maintaining his receptivity to ideas, knowledge and his own senses, thus providing the way for his inner forces and faculties to flow in a creative manner. To borrow from the Zen philosopher von Dürckheim (1980):

"The destiny of everything that lives is that is should unfold its own nature to its maximum possibility. He is only permitted to become fully what he is intended to be when he takes himself in hand, works on himself, and practices ceaselessly to reach perfection. It is evident that the prerequisites for this to succeed are: a mind completely at the service of the work in hand, a tenacious will, a capacity to assimilate the necessary experience, the efficient development of relevant talents and their proper techniques and, in addition to all this, the ability to achieve a continuous adaptation to the exterior world."

The role and function of the voice: an overview 5

The first four chapters of this book have emphasized the energy field, the whole singer, and how to bring some necessary changes to vocal pedagogy. At the same time, the most obvious aspects of the voice are those that are seen and heard. It is understandable that the first observations of voice professionals are related to the things they know well—physical structure and acoustic properties. These form an important foundation from which to explore the less audible and visible aspects of the human voice, and are important to all voice professionals and students. However, it is prudent to note that the physical and acoustic aspects are often symptoms of the non-physical and/or problems, and not the main source. At some point, it is worth knowing that for solving many problems, the voice professional will need to investigate the less obvious.

The voice is considered to be as much as thirty-eight percent of a person's communication when in combination with visible or non-verbal aspects (55%), and the words (7%). When speaking on the phone that percentage goes up enormously. When these elements are balanced and driven by core singing or speaking, there is a powerful, cohesive message. The balance of these elements will vary with the knowledge, maturity, and self-image, and perceptions of each student.

Communication

As the voice is usually an integral part of a singer's self-perception, it is always wise to consider the whole person rather than isolate the production of sound from personality. There are a number of key factors that relate the voice to the whole personality. The first is the broad area of communication (Fig. 1), which includes imparting information by use of language, communicating with a group or an individual, and specialised communication through performance. Thoughts and ideas are conveyed through choice of words, by tone of voice that is pleasant or unpleasant, gentle or harsh, by the rhythm that is inherent within the language itself and by personal speech rhythms that are flowing and regular, or uneven and hesitant, and finally, by the pitch and melody of the utterance. When speaking in public the voice may indicate lack of confidence or fright, confidence or calm and at interpersonal levels the tone may reflect ideas and feelings over and above the words chosen, or may belie them. Ultimately it is difficult to hide the way we feel because

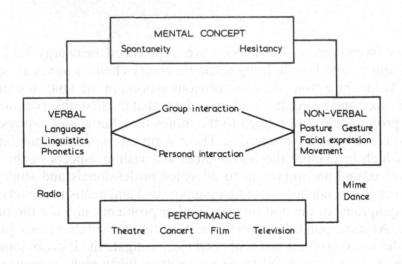

Fig. 1. Aspects of communication.
Communication for performance begins with the mental concept of what is to be presented. The concept includes verbal and non-verbal factors, both of which are also involved in interactions between groups and individuals. Not all types of performance include verbal and non-verbal factors, for example radio broadcasting is entirely dependent upon verbal impact and mime on visual impressions.

the listener will, consciously or unconsciously, detect in the sound intuitive sympathy or antipathy, lack of concern or interest, fatigue, anxiety, enthusiasm or excitement.

Enthusiasm and a desire to perform are key ingredients for appearing in public. Public performance can be a manner of communication that is highly specialised with its own techniques for obtaining effects by voice and/or gesture. However, personal motivation and that derived from the text, and the music (in the case of singing), in combination with the performer's skills, personality and ability to create empathy will determine the success of communication at artistic, political or pedagogic levels.

Psychological factors

Second, the voice gives psychological clues to a person's self-image (Fig. 2), perception of others and emotional health. Self-image can be indicated by a tone of voice that is confident, pretentious, shy, aggressive, outgoing, exuberant, to name only a few personality traits. In addition the sound may give a clue to the facade or mask of that person, for example a shy person hiding behind an over-confident front. How one perceives another person's receptiveness, interest or sympathy in

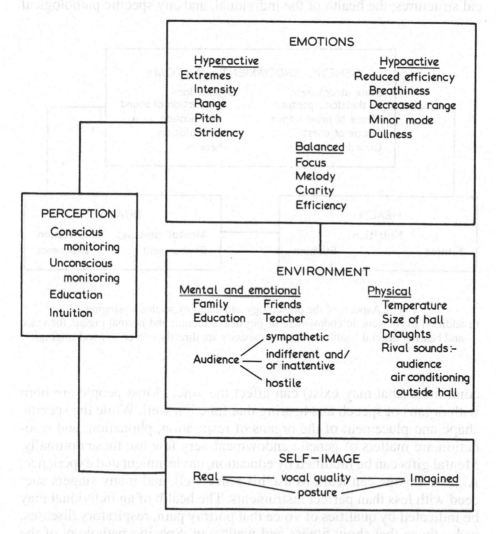

Fig. 2. Aspects of the psychology of voice and singing.
The use of the human voice includes the perception of the singer or speaker and the relation of their perception to the interrelated factors of emotion, environment and self-image.

any given conversation can drastically alter the tone of presentation, by encouraging or discouraging the speaker. Emotional health is evidenced in the voice by free and melodic sounds of the happy, by constricted and harsh sounds of the angry, and by dull and lethargic qualities in the depressed.

Physiological factors

Third, the physiological factors (Fig. 3) of genetic endowment of physical structures, the health of the individual, and any specific pathological

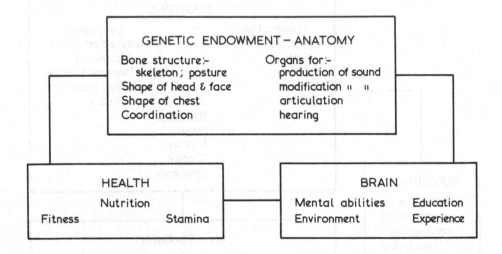

Fig. 3. Aspects of the physiology and anatomy related to singing.
In addition to the genetic endowment of physical structure and normal organs for voice and hearing general health and mental capacity are directly related to good singing.

conditions (that may exist) can affect the voice. Most people are born with organs of speech and hearing that function well. While the specific shape and placement of the organs of respiration, phonation, and resonation are matters of genetic endowment very few use these optimally. Mental gifts can be modified by education, environment and experience. Almost anyone can learn to use his voice well, and many singers succeed with less than perfect instruments. The health of an individual may be indicated by qualities of voice that portray pain, respiratory diseases, or by those that show fitness and wellbeing. Specific pathology of the vocal organs is usually revealed by hoarseness, roughness or lack of clarity in the sound.

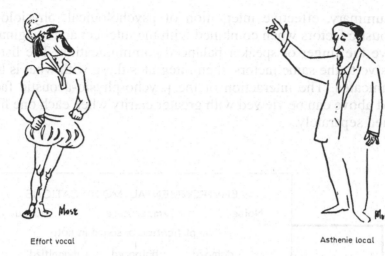

Effort vocal   Asthenie local

Fig. 4. Caricatures of singers who demonstrate excessive tension and lack of vocal energy. (As depicted in *La Voix,* 1953 by kind permission of Librairie Maloine, Paris.) These caricatures represent the image that the general public has of the typical opera singer, and of one type of singer of popular music. Many non-singers, and sometimes singers, associate operatic singing with excessive expenditure of energy because there are too many examples of these unfortunate mannerisms.

Note: the excessive opening of the mouth with resultant tension in the lips and jaw, protrusion of the jaw, the tight neck, rigidly braced shoulders and chest, arched back and locked knees. Popular singers go from one extreme to another, never still for a moment or so casual that they epitomize slackness and inertia as depicted here. The eyes are almost closed, the head tucked into the chest, the slouch is evidenced by rounded shoulders and protruding abdomen.

Acoustic and environmental factors

Fourth, acoustic factors (Fig. 5) such as auditory discrimination and hearing are important in influencing vocal production because fine modulation of sound partly depends on the discrimination and acuity of the hearing mechanism.

Environmental factors, in the broadest sense, play a considerable role in how a person uses his voice. These include acoustic, physical and social environments. Depending upon the perceptions and actual state of the performer, the acoustic environment of a room or concert hall, whether it is adequate, too live or too dead, and such physical factors as temperature, humidity, smoke and noise, can affect the quality of sound. The psychological environment, for example that between teacher and pupil, and the influence of the family, the degree of encouragement of proper speech habits, practice of the arts, music and reading can generate either a positive or negative influence on the potential artist.

In summary, effective integration of psychological, physiological and acoustic factors when combined with the intellect and imagination, will give the singer or speaker balanced communication. The listener, responsive to the same factors, then integrates these with what is being communicated. The interaction of the psycho-physio-acoustic factors outlined above can be viewed with greater clarity when each one first is examined separately.

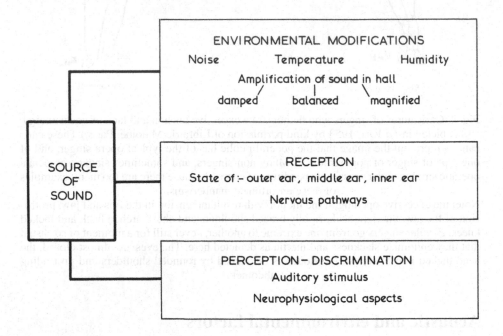

Fig. 5. Acoustic factors of singing.
The singer producing the sound, and the sound produced are both subject to environmental modification. The reception by the performer and audience is dependent upon the mechanism of hearing, and the acuity of perception and discrimination.

Psychological factors of communication

Moses (1954) and Rousey (1974) have written interesting treatises on psychology in relation to the use of the voice. They emphasise that emotion can be shown in the voice through different parameters such as breathing patterns and rhythm of utterance, pitch and speed, and distinctiveness of articulation.

Much of the time these patterns are perceived at the subconscious level. Almost anyone can sense when a friend is not feeling well from

his tone of voice. Even in a telephone conversation the untrained listener will respond to mood changes that are revealed by variations in
pitch levels and rhythm of speech. Emotion is reflected in the tempo of
speech: anxiety, excitement, anger and happiness tend to speed up the
tempo and rhythm; depression and undue stress slow it down.

A person's self-image and concept (Fig. 2) of what he says play extremely important roles in influencing his vocal quality and speech behaviour. A positive self-image is usually reflected in good posture and
carriage (head held high and back straight), and in confident speech that
is clear and precise. An insecure person can exhibit poor posture (slump-
ing shoulders and lowered head) and tends to mumble or speaks inau-
dibly. As Brodnitz (1953) and Moses (1954) also noted, a person's self-
image may influence the pitch of his voice: a case in point is the man
who is careful to speak in the deep register, or the woman who chooses
to retain a "little girl" high pitched sound.

A speaker's or singer's perception of the sound he is making differs
from the listener's perception of that sound (see Chapter 5), and it is
sometimes difficult to convince young singers and voice therapy patients that this is true. Sound of laryngeal origin is modified in the pharynx and in other supra-laryngeal regions, and as individuals we become
used to this sound and consider it to be part of our own image or being.
Often when singers or speakers hear their voices on a tape recorder for
the first time, they initially reject the sound as representing their true
selves. It can be disturbing when one realises that what others hear is
different, particularly when the sound is perceived as representing one's
self-image and personality. In some cases a teacher will have trouble
implementing a change in tonal quality because the student incorrectly
feels he is being asked to change his personality. When a student can
be persuaded that the goal is to *sense* the sound rather than to hear and
judge according to old, unreliable criteria, the teacher will probably be
successful in any effort to obtain vocal modification. When the singer
has the added advantage of video feedback, the task becomes much easier.

There are many subjective terms for various voice qualities – nasal,
warm, pleasant, vibrant, strident, breathy, harsh – and each of these terms
may indicate a distinct psychological or physiological state. A voice that
is consistently strident indicates excessive tension in the speaker or singer. Listeners will usually react with a sympathetic throat ache or feeling
of discomfort, and, in the case of the singer, this can even happen to an
audience. Hence, much of a listener's perception of what is being said
can be based on his sympathetic response to the quality of the sound,
rather than on the actual meaning of the words. Therefore it is important
for a speaker or singer to understand the choice of sounds available in

his own voice so that he will not create a double message with unintended qualities or inflections which appear to negate the words.

Physiological factors

Any study of the physiology of vocal production (Fig.3) will reveal the
complexity of the various anatomical parts and the intricate co-ordination needed for these parts to produce sounds. All musical instruments
have an initial energy that activates the vibrator, the vibrator itself, and
a resonator. The physical instrument for human sound production and
has as its activator the breath or respiratory system; a primary vibrator, the vocal folds; and a resonator consisting of the upper part of the
larynx and mouth, (also the nose for some sounds) with the intervening
pharynx being the most important of all. The singer, unlike inanimate
musical instruments, has one additional and very important element: ar-
ticulator structures for forming words. Despite Anna Russell's (1952)
statement that *"singers have resonance where their brains ought to be,"*
the singer has a brain to activate and control all these elements, and a
dynamic postural structure to form a supporting framework for them.

Briefly, vocal sound is created as follows. (This process is analysed
in detail in Chapter 7). Air from the lungs flows through the glottis causing the vocal folds to vibrate; the pharynx then resonates, intensifies
and modifies these vibrations; and finally words are added by means of
the structures of articulation. These structures also have other functions
to perform and can prove antagonistic to the processes of singing and
speaking. Therefore, teachers and students of voice need to be familiar
with both functions of the components of vocal production in order to
make accurate analyses. The chapters that follow will expand and clarify
this point.

Some important and relevant physiological studies have been con-
ducted in humans by Bouhuys (1966, 1968), Proctor (1968, 1980) and
Leanderson (1987, 1988) on breathing; Faaborg-Andersen (1967) and
Vennard (1971) made electromyographic studies of the activity of musculature of the vocal folds and Kirchner and Wyke (1964) and Wyke and
Kirchner (1976) investigated the neurophysiology of the larynx. (See
Chapter 7 for specific details). However, bear in mind that some aspects
of research of this sort are understandably limited by a singer's reactions
to performing while attached to unfamiliar measuring devices.

The primary breathing apparatus consists of the diaphragm, lungs,
rib cage, the muscles responsible for enlarging the thorax for inspiration
or diminishing it for expiration, and the abdominal muscles. A detailed

physiological analysis of breathing is provided in Chapter 6. However there is also a psychological component to the breathing process that is of interest. As indicated earlier, breathing patterns can give clues to personality and feelings. Moses (1954) noted that shallow-rapid breathing showed excitement or agitation, and slow controlled breathing denoted calmness and confidence. An extremely tense or excited person will have shallow (high chest) breathing patterns, or seem not to breath at all, and will run out of breath in the middle of sentences and phrases. By contrast, an angry person will manifest intensity by taking very few breaths and by running sentences together. The person who is balanced in his speech and his emotions breathes deeply and evenly. Breathing patterns are used as diagnostic tests in various diseased states such as emphysema where the patient has trouble breathing out, has inadequate oxygen exchange and is therefore breathless in conversation. Thus he is not able to sustain sound for more than a few (3–5) seconds. By contrast, a healthy person is likely to continue for at least 30 seconds; a sustained vowel such as /i/ (meet) will probably last as long as 15 seconds.

The primary phonatory mechanism or vibrator consists of the vocal folds and auxiliary muscles housed in and about the larynx. The closing of these folds to initiate sound, commonly called the "attack" or onset in vocal instruction, is controlled by a number of factors: the amount of pressure generated by exhalation, the physical tension in the larynx, subglottic pressure (see Chapter 7), and the intent or concept of the desired sound as conceived by the speaker or singer. Personality, physiological state and concept of sound all have an effect on the activity of laryngeal muscles. Tense people usually exhibit excessive muscular constriction in the throat and can create a sound that has an unpleasant, strident quality making the listener uncomfortable without realising the reason. Other forms of tension may be manifested by excessive clearing of the throat or swallowing before speaking. By contrast, people who tend to be lax suffer from a slow, inefficient muscular co-ordination and typically produce a vocal attack that is excessively breathy, unclear or imprecise.

The resonation of vocal sound takes place mainly in the pharynx. A musical instrument has a solid or fixed resonator as in the body of a violin, clarinet or piano. However the pharynx is an adjustable, mobile, muscular sleeve that can assume many changes of shape and variations of tension in its walls. These adjustments are governed by the imagination which influences the adjustment of the muscles of the pharynx to produce different vocal qualities.

The pharynx is divided into nasal, oral and laryngeal sections, and each of the three sections contributes to resonance. The oral pharynx is the most adjustable area because of the mobility of the tongue and soft palate. The laryngeal pharynx is thought to contribute the "singer's formant" (Chapter 8), the reinforced overtone area which gives the good singer the proper carrying power to sing over the orchestra and to sing unaided by a microphone in large halls. The nasal pharynx contributes nasal resonance, considered undesirable except for certain sounds such as some in the French language, and in speech patterns in some countries, as well as in regional dialects in some countries like the United States of America and Australia. Specific areas and structures contributing to resonance will be discussed in detail in Chapter 8.

Emotional problems and tensions may manifest themselves as types of disease, however they are more likely to be present in the quality of the voice (Fig. 4). Tension in the pharynx manifests in rigid and constricted muscles, leaving little resonating space. This small amount of space coupled with the muscular tension that creates the rigidity can result in sounds that are strident, harsh or "white", and pinched or driven.

The various shapes of the pharynx also create a different coupling of the resonating areas and therefore alter the overtones in such a way as to change vocal quality. A slackness of muscle tone will create a sound that lacks intensity and may allow a nasal "honky" tone created by air escaping through the nose (because the palate is lowered). In addition, tongue tension can cause changes in the oral pharynx as well as create a sound that is garbled. Many of these tensions are seen in the physiological and acoustic patterns of regional characteristics ("accent") and result in the nasal twang, broad vowel sounds, or exaggerated r's attributed to certain geographical areas. It is common for particular types of lip movements and certain patterns of sound to run in families. Phoneticians can readily identify these differences. Because such speech differences exist, the teacher of singing must know the standard pronunciation for the languages used in opera and recital repertoire, and in regional dialect for contemporary commercial music so that proper changes in sound can be effected readily.

Acoustic factors

We are able to measure the acoustic or audible aspects of voice with sophisticated equipment. The voice print analyser, sonograph, glottograph, airflow meter, pressure recorder and computerised models of the vocal tract enable investigators to confirm earlier empirical findings and unearth new aspects of vocal sound characterisation. The physiological aspects of sound production such as breathing patterns, vocal attack, vocal fold vibration, and some resonance qualities can be revealed and substantiated by acoustic means. Just such experiments have been performed by several researchers including Winckel (1952/53), Ladefoged (1962b), Sundberg (1973, 1987), and Cleveland (1977) and many others who have used spectral analysers to study and record vocal tract resonances or formants.[1]

The study of vocal acoustics is one of the most attractive and least invasive ways of investigating the voice. More information about this valuable area of research can be found in the work of Titze (1994), Sundberg (1987), both respected and tireless investigators.

Less studied is the area of acoustic feedback, psychologically and empirically, a critical area for any singer.

Perception

Machines are important tools for laboratory research, however for purposes of performance and the teaching of singing, the human ear (see Berendt, 1988) and associated neural mechanisms provide a superb instrument for refined detection and analysis of sound (Fig. 5). Such analysis has given rise to considerable research in psychology. For example, in 1936 Seashore wrote about music as follows:

"Between the physical world of vibration as measured by apparatus, and the world of consciously heard music, there is a third area of investigation. Our auditory apparatus and/or mind separates different instruments and tones, hears pleasantness and unpleasantness, establishes sensations of volume, hears some vibrations however not others, adds tones to fill out the sound spectrum, etc. This middle ground is the province of the psychology of music, a subject about which even the physical scientists know little."

Today the psychologists refer to this "third area of investigation" as

---

[1] Ladefoged (1962) has defined formants as follows: "The peaks in the spectrum of vowels correspond to the basic frequencies of the vibration of the air in the vocal tract. The region of the spectrum in which the frequency corresponds are relatively large and known as formants. The formants of a sound are those aspects of it which are directly dependent on the shape of the vocal tract, and are largely responsible for the characteristic quality ... It is the presence of formants that enables us to recognise the different vowels which are associated with the different positions of the vocal organ."

studies in perception and musical ability; and there is considerable interest in modes of hearing music, the neuro-physiological processes involved and the possibility of accurately assessing musicality. Studies by Smith and Burkland (1966) regarding the specific hemispheres of the brain concerned with singing, and those of Kimura (1964) with respect to primary perception of melody by the right or left ear have led to interesting speculations about the functioning of the brain in relation to musical tasks.

A compilation of such studies can be found in 'Music and the Brain' edited by Critchley and Henson (1977) and in 'Music, Mind and Brain edited by Clynes (1982). The articles contained in these books are fascinating perhaps with more questions being asked than answered. Maria Wyke (1977) has suggested that two important points emerge:

1. That patterns of cerebral specialisation may be different for the perception of the components of musical talent;
2. Patterns of cerebral specialisation and hemispheric interaction may be different for musically sophisticated and musically naive subjects. In future we may have some informative answers to such questions as well as some practical means of assessing musical talent.[2]

Musical perception includes the intuitive recognition of the aesthetic qualities of music. There are three fundamentally important aspects of the act of perceiving: the first is a person's ability to hear accurately with no impairment of the anatomical structures of the hearing mechanism; the second phase of perception is the actual stimulation of the sensory receptor systems of the ear; and the third concerns the neuro-physiological aspects. In addition, one has to include the roles of emotion, intellect and education in the perceptual processes.

The teacher of singing has the responsibility of educating the performer and the listener and therefore must cultivate accurate perceptions. To that end a necessary requisite for the teacher is a keen analytical ability enabling accurate interpretation of the responses of the ear to variance in

---

[2] Although there are a number of tests which assess musical ability, their validity as overall measurements of talent has been seriously questioned. It is possible to demonstrate the ability of a person to recognise and understand changes in musical and quasi-musical tests, but assessment of specific musical abilities has been largely unsuccessful (Shuter, 1968). One of the reasons for this is that the measurement of musical ability has been hampered by the lack of agreement on the nature of musical skill (M. Wyke, 1977). For further comment on musical testing, see Wing (1941), McLeish (1950) and Shuter (1968).

rhythm, pitch and qualities of voice. Because the perception of sound by the listener is a very important factor in aesthetic judgement, the teacher must be able to draw from a student those tones and qualities which are vocally healthy and pleasing to the ear.

Teachers' analytical ability in combination with their education and intuition will enable the establishment of a common ground from which to work with the student. The physiological, acoustic, psychological, and mental aspects of singing will form the basis for shared perceptions and a foundation from which to enjoy the study of singing or voice. What remains now, is to look at the remarkable physical structures that make up the human voice.

6 Posture and breathing in singing

Posture and physical alignment

The structure and alignment of the human skeleton is the scaffolding on which all other parts of the body depend. Therefore any discussion of the vocal mechanism must begin here. Posture, mental attitude, and genetic propensity determine the alignment and balance of the body, and good bodily alignment is the beginning of efficient breathing and fundamental to healthy singing.

In this era of the casual, it is rare to see someone with proper physical poise (Fig. 6). Young children with poor posture are often not corrected; and adolescents – and even adults – are anxious to blend in with stoop-shouldered peers. Sitting at computers has contributed to the problem as well. However, singers, actors, and dancers cannot survive profession-ally unless they can choose and govern their posture precisely. There-fore teachers of the performing arts must correct the bad postural habits of a generation of slouchers. The task of changing habits is formidable, however proper alignment improves health, performance and one's self-image. For centuries Oriental thinking and philosophy have stressed the interdependence of mind and body (see von Durchheim, 1977); physical alignment and balance being fundamentally linked with mental balance and peace within one's self. In the West this concept is gradually being absorbed. To any performing artist, mental and physical balance and agil-ity are important, however the first is beyond the scope of this discussion which is concerned with physical balance, an essential asset for singing.

Basmajian (1978) has said that the balance of the erect human body depends on a delicate neutralization of forces of gravity. In other words, a person is posturally well-balanced when he can stand, walk and sit without a pronounced increase in muscular activity. Those with poor posture are balanced as they sit, stand and walk or they could not be upright, however this is only at an unnecessary cost of muscular activ-ity and energy. A singer cannot afford to waste energy on faulty posture during performance.

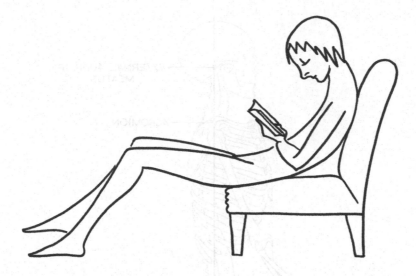

Fig. 6. The casual posture.
Although at first sight this may appear relaxed, it involves a large amount of muscular stress, particularly on the back and neck. In addition, movement of the cramped chest is restricted and the pull of gravity on the head has to be counteracted by muscles on the back of the neck.

Gould (1971) emphasizes that posture is the dynamic inter-relationship between muscular and skeletal tissues. The word dynamic is important because it implies a stable alignment rather than one that is static and fixed, and it is a prelude to easy, flowing movement. It takes extra muscular to change a fixed posture, thus leaving a feeling of bodily heaviness. When postural alignment is dynamic, a feeling of lightness and ease of movement ensues.

The body is aligned efficiently when a plumb line can be shown to fall from the top of the head through the ear hole (external auditory meatus) the middle of the point of the shoulder (acromion), the highest point on the iliac crest, the knees, and just in front of the ankle. Figure 7 demonstrates very clearly the correct postural alignment of the skeleton. Note the following:

a) The head is up, face forward, and the external auditory meatus is vertically above the middle of the point of the shoulder.
b) The chest is high, yet not rigid as in a military position of attention.
c) The highest point of the pelvis is also on the same line (as the external auditory meatus and acromion).

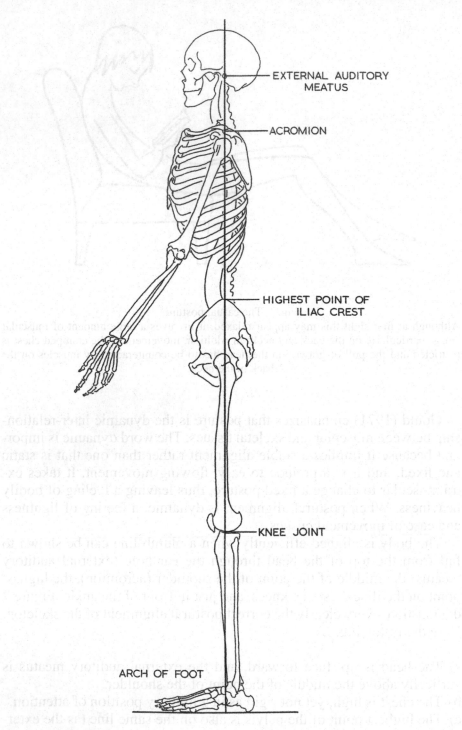

Fig. 7. Balanced posture depicted by a line drawing of the human skeleton.

d) When standing in a good posture with the feet together or slightly apart, the line from the ear and shoulder continues through the knee joint and in front of the ankle. The knees are not braced back rigidly. In walking, the upper part of the torso is balanced comfortably over, not in front of the legs and feet.

e) With such an alignment the natural curves of the vertebral column are preserved while it remains poised and not braced, and therefore there is minimal muscular activity. The movements of the spine are constantly and rhythmically altered in stance, walking and running, in order to maintain balance.

For many years physiologists have shown that the position of the head on the neck is vital because it governs all postural reflexes. When the head is misaligned other parts of the body move in or out of line to maintain balance and thus energy is expended to counteract the effect of gravity. A review of studies by Wyke (review 1979a, b) have shown that the mechanoreceptors[1] in the area around the joints and joint capsules of the cervical region have an influence on gait and posture. Therefore any changes in position of the head can affect postural muscles of the limbs and chest, a point to be remembered by singers who have to move about on stage.

Because multiple adjustments are required to stabilize the body against gravity, (Fig. 8), faulty posture of any part of the body leads to misalignment. Some typical problems teachers will see and have to correct are improper position of the head, rounded shoulders, a cramped chest, and excessively arched lower back (lordosis) and locked knees. A head poked forward in hurrying from place to place will be associated with compensatory arching of the back and an abnormal position of the pelvis. Even stationary performers may talk or sing with their heads or chins jutting forwards. This is not only unsightly; it interferes with the proper positioning of the pharynx for singing and speaking (see Chapters 8 and 9).

Bracing the shoulders and chest wastes energy and surprisingly, the seemingly relaxed posture of rounded shoulders is also tiring. Round shoulders are unsightly, hamper the movements of the chest, and are acquired by slouching in chairs and poor standing posture. Many do

---

[1] Mechanoreceptors are specialized nerve endings sensitive to alterations of stretch and pressure. They are found in deeper parts of skin, muscles, tendons, capsules and ligaments of joints. When activated these receptors send coded messages by electrical impulses into the central nervous system to control mustcular activity reflexly in respone to changes in muscular activity itself and/or the position of joints.

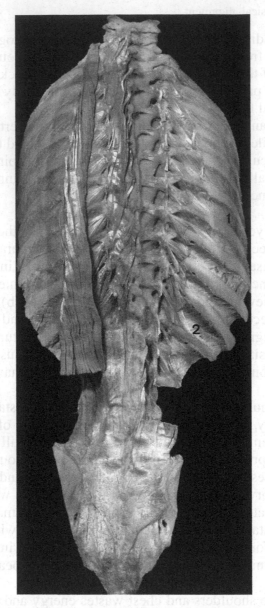

Fig. 8. Dissection of the back of the lower cervical region, thorax, lumbar and sacral vertebral column.

(By kind permission of the Anatomy Department of the Royal College of Surgeons of England.) A. Some of the muscles controlling the vertebral column are shown on the left side. Note their complexity, massiveness, and the different attachments and orientations of their fibers which affect their directions of pull. This post-vertebral group has a profoundly important postural function. Balanced activity between the abdominal muscles and those in the lumbar region control the movements and curves of the spine other than the cervical and sacral ones. Any persisting asymmetrical pull results in abnormal curves of the spine with shortening of ligaments and even alterations in shapes of bones. B. On the right side note the fibers of the external intercostal muscles (1), and the internal intercostal membrane is seen in the lower spaces (2).

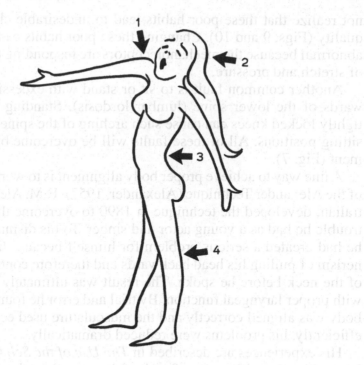

Fig. 9. Poor postural habits of a singer who is "carried away".
Singers who labor their technique and/or the emotions of the music often develop unconscious postural habits which detract from their appearance and inhibit fine singing. In this
caricature note: the tensely raised shoulder (1), the head is thrown back (2), the back is
arched and the abdomen protruded (3), and the knees locked (4).

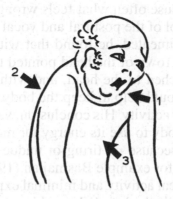

Fig. 10. The "inward" singer.
The face is expressionless, the chin tucked into the neck (1), the shoulders are rounded (2)
and chest cramped (3).

not realize that these poor habits lead to undesirable changes in vocal quality (Figs. 9 and 10). Changing these poor habits can feel strange or abnormal because the mechanoreceptors are responding to a new pattern of stretch and pressure.

Another common fault is to sit or stand with excessive arching forwards of the lower spine (lumbar lordosis). Standing with braced or tightly locked knees can cause such arching of the spine, as can certain sitting positions. All of these faults will be overcome by correct alignment (Fig. 7).

A fine way to achieve proper body alignment is to work with a teacher of the Alexander Technique (Alexander, 1957). F. M. Alexander, an Australian, developed the technique in 1890 to overcome the serious vocal trouble he had as a young actor and singer. To his dismay he found that he had created a serious problem for himself because he had the mannerism of pulling his head backwards and therefore contracting muscles of the neck before he spoke. The result was ultimately an interference with proper laryngeal function. By trial and error he found that when his body was aligned correctly and the musculature used economically and efficiently, his problems were reduced dramatically.

His experiences are described in *The Use of the Self* (1946), and it is interesting that although at first he felt correctly poised, he found that his posture and habits were incorrect. By experiment he learned to align his head and body so that long standing reflexes and habits were broken. With new alignment came the understanding that his old concepts of posture and of use of his voice resulted from misdirection of his body. Initially the correct alignment felt very awkward and even wrong. This concept of what feels right or wrong is important to posture and to the process of singing because often what feels wrong or unusual at first is actually physical control of the postural and vocal mechanisms.

As Alexander experimented, he found that with the head held high as if floating, with the crown of the head pointed to the ceiling, and the spine like a string attached to the head, and with the arms and shoulders relaxed, gravity would help to keep the body in alignment with no need for great muscular activity. His conclusion was that this freedom of alignment allows the body to use its energy far more economically and is especially efficient because no tiring or undue tensions are present. Functional anatomists, for example Basmajian (1978), have shown that there is minimal electrical activity and minimal expenditure of energy in postural muscles when the body is balanced in correct alignment.

The Alexander Technique is taught by verbal and tactile suggestions gently guiding the student into the use of his muscles and the proper positioning of his body. The pupil is helped to feel and recognize sensations of proper positions of the body until correct habits in sitting, standing, and walking are developed and become spontaneous and dynamic. As thorough and analytical examination of each individual is required, teachers of this technique are certified only after three years of study at specified centers or with authorized teachers. Tinbergen paid tribute to the Alexander Technique and the value of such para-medical teaching in his acceptance speech for the Nobel Prize in Physiology and Medicine in 1974. He and his family had reaped beneficial results from such teaching.

Respiration

Breathing seems to be a simple process, one that requires no thought. However subconscious reflex control of respiration is complicated and delicately adjusted to the needs of the body. In addition to supplying the body with oxygen and removing carbon dioxide, breathing generates all vocal sound. Normally one does not have to think about breathing for conversational speech, yet during performance one becomes quite conscious of the need for adequate and efficient control of breath.

Medical science has been concerned with the normal physiology, diseases and specific pathological conditions in relation to respiration, and with normal respiration in athletes at high altitudes or using underwater apparatus. The finer points of professional voice production, whether singing or the varied forms of speech, have not been studied in detail from a scientific standpoint, or with any sizable number of subjects. Campbell (1969, 1970) and Newsom Davis and Sears (1970) have made valuable studies of the function of respiratory muscles (see Wyke, 1974 for review). As the body of scientific literature about respiration increases, so do the discrepancies in conclusions reached. One reason is that investigators assume that all their subjects are using a common pattern of breathing. The other is that scientists are often contradicted by teachers of singing, who have adhered to a tradition that has been handed down from one generation to another. As a result, there are almost as many techniques of breathing as there are performers; and the researchers and teachers are not seeing any uniformity of performance. Instead they are observing a compendium of personal experience, idiosyncracies, and to add to the problem, are using a confusing terminology.

Despite the contradictions, this research provides a basis from which further more objective studies can proceed. Even now there is much of value for the teachers who wish to use an informed and reasoned approach when coaching students in the process of breathing. This chapter discusses posture and breathing in the light of results of current research, analysis of singing techniques, and observation of normal and abnormal breathing patterns in singers, actors, athletes, and patients with respiratory disorders and diseases.

Quiet respiration

Quiet respiration, which occurs at rest or during minimal bodily activity, requires little physical energy and is a reflex action. The mechanism is as follows: (1) a message from the brain causes the diaphragm to contract, thus enlarging the thorax; (2) this enlargement of the chest pulls on the lungs causing a big drop in the pressure of the lungs in relation to the pressure of the atmosphere (this can occur because the lungs and thoracic air passages are formed largely of elastic tissue) and air is sucked in to counteract the tendency to form a vacuum-like condition; (3) during expiration the diaphragm relaxes, and the lungs, elastic air passages and the chest wall recoil. The process of quiet respiration is repeated about seventeen times per minute in a healthy adult at rest, with an intake of approximately 500ml of air. For stage performance more air, and therefore, more physical energy, are necessary, and efficient breathing must initially become a conscious or voluntary act. Proctor (1980) writes, *"It is immediately apparent that gross alterations in the pattern of quiet breathing are necessary for phonation. During speech the greater portion of air flow passes through the mouth rather than the nose: inspirations are brief and rapid; expirations are prolonged and slow; and airway pressures are more negative in inspiration and more positive in expiration. These variances from ordinary breathing are more pronounced in singing than in speaking."* Because these variations are so pronounced in singing, the efficient co-ordination of respiratory mechanisms is fundamental to good vocal production. Correct breathing for singing may have to be practised consciously when the singer's habits inhibit efficient vocal production. Ultimately these movements are automatically programmed and become reflex. The good singer subconsciously judges and uses the amount of air needed in every song for each phrase regardless of the length (for discussion see Wyke, 1979). When movement is controlled reflexly, conscious effort can then be focused on interpretation rather than on mechanics of singing.

Singers often focus their attention on the expiration of breath since much of their music demands lengthy phrases and prolonged control of release of air. However, efficient inspiration provides the correct physiological setting for efficient expiration, and therefore both aspects of the breathing process must be discussed.

Inspiration

In singing, the most efficient inspiration is one that allows the desired amount of air to be drawn in rapidly and inconspicuously without inducing undue muscular interference with the functioning of the lips, tongue, jaw, pharynx and larynx. During inspiration the lungs expand by means of enlargement of every dimension of the thorax, which may be accomplished by several groups of muscles, some of which bear the main responsibility for the action (prime movers). Some other muscles aid inspiration in extreme effort, and are not usually important to singing. They are known as accessory muscles of respiration. Other secondary muscles are those in which limited contraction helps to stabilize the rib cage and/or aid in posture without interfering with efficient inspiration. In extreme conditions, which should never be encountered in singing, all these muscles may be responding. They are listed in anatomy texts and are irrelevant in this discussion. To understand the way respiratory muscles work it is necessary to have some knowledge of the bony skeleton upon which they act (Figs. 11, 12, 13).

The orientation and length of the ribs and the shape and orientation of the joints between ribs, vertebrae and sternum govern the direction and ranges through which the ribs can move. When ribs 1–5 are moved during inspiration they increase the anterior-posterior (AP) diameter of the chest (Fig. 14). These ribs are often described as having a pump-handle motion. The well-trained singer does not move these very much for two reasons; (1) the diaphragm plays a major role in their breathing pattern and (2) the rib cage is already partially elevated by the assumption of correct posture. Excessive movement of these ribs during inspiration is detrimental to singing because it usually involves the action of neck muscles which pull up the upper two ribs and sternum to which they are attached. The size of the chest is increased laterally and somewhat anterior-posteriorly by the movement of ribs 5, 6 and 7. Because ribs 8–10 are directly attached to the costal cartilage of the 7th rib they also participate in this movement. This action is often described as bucket-handle (Fig. 15). When the body is properly aligned, these natural movements[2] of the lower chest and abdomen become obvious both to the singer and trained observer.

Inspection of the skeletal elements of the thorax shows that the thoracic cavity is curiously shaped. The base of this cavity is formed by the diaphragm, a large domed, muscle, which separates the thorax and abdomen. The gaps between the ribs are filled in by intercostal muscles and membranes; the top of each half of the cavity is covered in by a dome of tough fibrous material (fascia). The cavity related to the lungs is lined

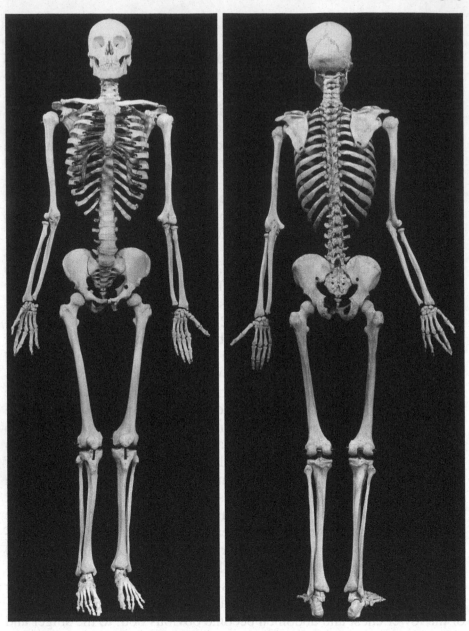

Fig. 11. Bony skeleton – anterior view.   Fig. 12. Bony skeleton – posterior view.

Figs. 11 and 12 show the entire skeleton, but particular attention should be paid to the cervical and thoracic vertebral column, ribs, costal cartilages and sternum. There are twelve pairs of ribs, the first pair is attached to the sternum by bars of cartilage, the second to seventh pairs have a moveable synovial joint between the costal cartilage and sternum. The costal cartilages of the eighth to tenth ribs are attached to those of the seventh, and therefore, only indirectly to the sternum. The eleventh and twelfth have no sternal attach-

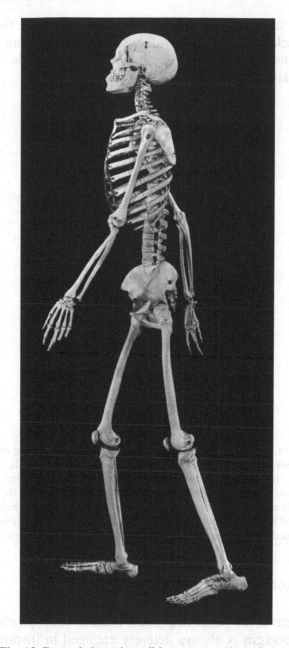

Fig. 13. Bony skeleton in walking posture – lateral view.

ment. These three groups of ribs are also known as true, false and floating respectively. The parts of a typical rib include the facet for attachment to the vertebra, the neck, angle and shaft.

(Figs. 11,12, and 13 by kind permission of the Departments of Anatomy and Photography of the Royal Free Hospital School of Medicine).

with a closed sac of a smooth, moist elastic membrane, the pleura (Fig. 16). The muscles forming the walls and floor of the thorax play a primary part in inspiration and those attached to the outside of the rib cage have a secondary role.

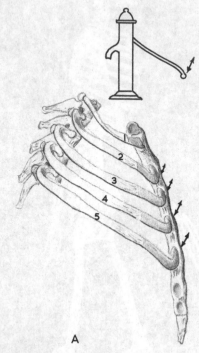

Fig. 14. Schematic representation of bucket handle motion of rips.
Note: The anterior ends of the ribs are lower than the posterior ends. The shape of the joints only allows for rotation, because of this and the slope noted above, the anterior ends move upwards and forwards, and downwards and backwards, hence the term pump handle movement. In addition these ribs are attached directly to the sternum. The change in the dimensions of the chest produced by movements of these shorter ribs is less than that produced by the more complex movements of the longer lower ones.

a) The diaphragm

The diaphragm is the most important muscle of inspiration (Figs. 17–20). The diaphragm is always actively engaged in inspiration. It is responsible for at least 60–80% of increased volume in deep inspiration. It is a large, double domed sheet of muscle with a central trefoil shaped tendon. When relaxed, the dome (the right dome is a little higher than the left) can ascend as high as the fifth intercostal space, which is much higher than is normally achieved in quiet or passive expiration. It should be noted that abdominal organs, for example the greater parts of the liver

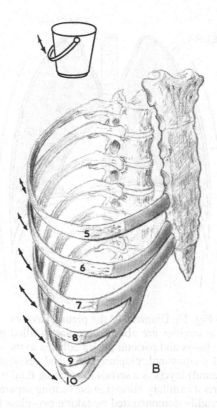

Fig. 15. Schematic representation of bucket handle motion of ribs.
The costo-vertebral joints of ribs of the fifth to tenth pairs allow anterior-posterior and lateral movement of these ribs. The eighth, ninth and tenth pairs are capable of considerable lateral movement because they have no direct attachment to the sternum, also the long bars of cartilage at the costal margin allow for considerable distortion during inspiratory movement, and the restoration of this deformation plays an important role in expiration during quiet respiration. It follows that calcification, and therefore hardening, of these cartilages which may occur with aging will limit freedom of respiratory movement.

and stomach, lie beneath the diaphragm and are largely protected by the rib cage. When the muscle contracts it flattens and comes forwards increasing the length, and therefore the capacity, of the thoracic cavity, thus allowing air to rush in. This flattening also pushes the abdominal organs downwards and forwards and creates a bulge in the epigastrium (upper abdomen). Many singers incorrectly believe this bulge is due to the diaphragm itself. Brodnitz (1954) suggested that this confusion would be reduced if the phrase "abdominal breathing" were used instead of the misleading phrase "diaphragmatic breathing". Both terms are correct as long as one realizes that it is diaphragmic movement displacing the abdominal organs that causes the bulge. However, "abdominal

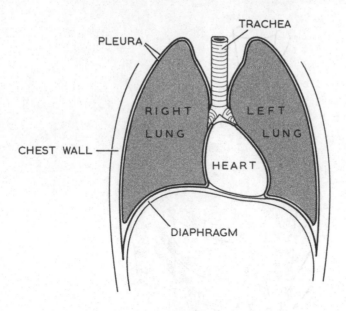

Fig. 16. Diagram of the pleural cavities.
The right and left pleural cavities are almost completely filled by lung. Visceral pleura covers the surface of the lungs and parietal pleura adheres to the walls of the pleural cavity which include costal mediastinal, diaphragmatic and cervical portions. Between the visceral and parietal (pleural) layers is a serous lubricating fluid which allows frictionless movement and also exerts a capillary attraction preventing separation of the visceral and parietal layers. This is readily demonstrated by taking two glass laboratory slides, moistening one and laying it on top of the other. They will glide easily in any direction but considerable force required to separate them. At the sternal borders and the periphery of the diaphragm parietal pleura forms recesses which are opened up during inspiration by the expansion of the lungs.

breathing" is probably the less confusing term.

Inspiration is always an active process requiring muscular contraction, while *quiet* expiration is purely passive, due to relaxation of the diaphragm and of the muscles, as well as elastic recoil of the lungs, trachea and cartilages of the thoracic cage. The amount of air used by a singer is considerably less than that used during athletic exercise or heavy manual work, however more than is required at rest. The needs of the singer lie somewhere between passive and forced breathing and may vary according to the music, dramatic situation, posture and the emotions of the performer. For example, the operatic singer who is forced to die on a couch while singing high C needs a great deal of air quickly. In this case the diaphragm and muscles of secondary importance may have to contract. Accessory muscles of inspiration ideally are not activated in singing (although they may be called on in respiratory distress) are not discussed here.

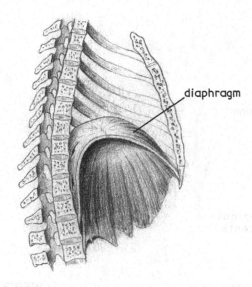

diaphragm

Fig. 17. Drawing of the left half of the diphram. (As seen from the side). *Note: The spine and sternum have been cut in half.* The diaphragm arises by two muscular slips (the crura or legs) from the first, second and third lumbar vertebrae on the right, and first and second on the left; from five so called ligaments which are tough fibrous arches; the lower border of the inner surfaces of the costal margin of the lower six ribs, and the back of the junction between the body and xiphoid process of the sternum. The muscular fibers curve upwards and are inserted into the central tendon.

b) The intercostal muscles

There are external, internal, and an incomplete innermost layer of intercostal muscles lying between the ribs (Figs. 21–23). These muscles maintain the stability of the chest wall and prevent it from being sucked in as the pressure falls inside the cavity during inspiration. In the past (and still found in many anatomy books) it was assumed that the external layer raised the ribs and was therefore inspiratory, and that the internal and innermost layers lowered the ribs and were therefore expiratory in function. The stabalizing role of these muscles is certain and any other role has been debated for years and is still controversial. Much of the literature on intercostal function in books relating to voice and speech is not up-to-date, so a short review of research is included here.

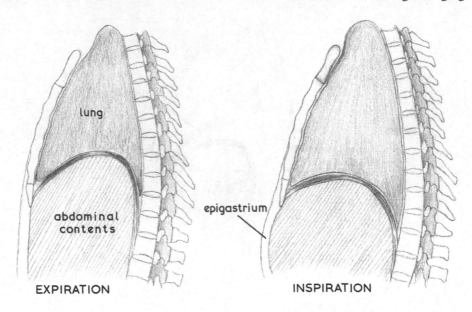

Fig. 18. Diagram of respiratory movements of the diaphragm.
During normal expiration the diaphragm is relaxed. On inspiration the muscle contracts
and increases the dimensions of the thorax from above downwards. This, coupled with
movements of ribs, causes visible forward displacement of the anterior chest wall and upper abdomen (epigastrium). Any deviation from this pattern of movement in people with
normal respiratory function may be due to habits of posture and/or training. In many singers and trained athletes quiet respiration is due almost entirely to diaphragmatic movement
and the rib cage is almost stationary. Dancers must keep the abdominal muscles contracted
for support of the vertebral column, therefore their breathing pattern results in movement
of the upper abdomen and lateral movement of the ribs with little movement of the lower
abdomen. On the contrary, one is likely to see much more abdominal excursion and less
anterior chest movement in singers.
(Note: the edges of the diaphragm and chest wall are in contact during expiration, but the
ribs and diaphragm peel apart during inspiration).

The electrical activity of contracting respiratory muscles was investigated by Campbell (1955, 1958) by means of surface electrodes. These
electrodes are placed on the skin overlying the muscle and and pick up
signals from a wide area and record the nearest muscle. He concluded
that some parts of the intercostals were active in quiet inspiration and in
voluntary forced expiration and that no distinction was possible between
the internal and external layers. This is not unexpected when surface
electrodes are employed. Taylor (1960) then made a study of the intercostals by means of special needle electrodes which could be inserted
directly in the muscles. This technique was more refined and enabled
him to record from a smaller area. His research was carried out on 80

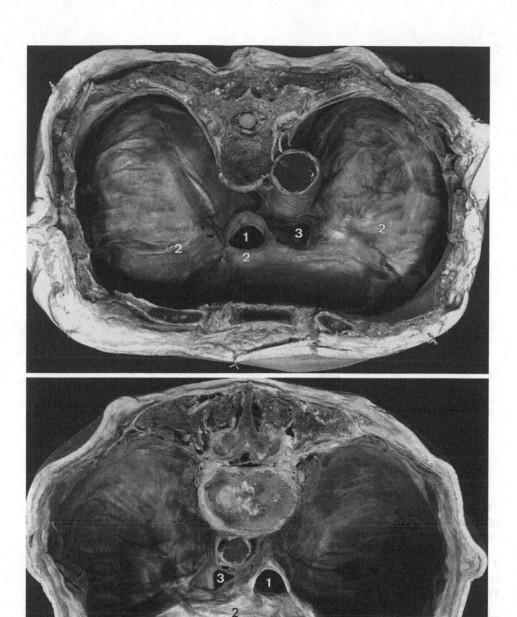

Fig. 19. (top) Superior surface of diaphragm.
Fig. 20. (bottom) Inferior surface of diaphragm.
(By kind permission of the Anatomy Department of the Royal College of Surgeons of England). Note: The thin walled inferior vena cava *(1)* is in the central tendon *(2)* and therefore held open widely during inspiration facilitating return of venous blood to the heart. The oesophagus *(3)* passes through muscle.

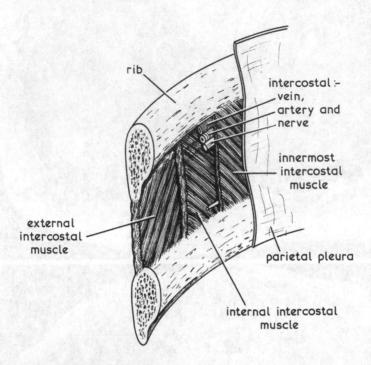

Fig. 21. Diagram of the intercostal muscles.

The *external intercostal* muscles extend from the tubercles of the ribs to the lateral borders of the costal cartilages. They are then continued as a thin sheet-like tendon (aponeurosis) called the external intercostal membrane. The muscle fibers slope obliquely downwards and forwards from the upper rib to the one below.

The *internal intercostal* muscles extend from the edge of the sternum or ends of the intercostal spaces to the postenor angles of the ribs and are then continued to the edge of the vertebral column as the internal intercostal membrane. Fibers slope obliquely downwards and backwards from the upper rib to the one below.

The *innermost intercostal* muscles lie deep to the internal intercostals and the fibers run in the same direction. This layer is composed of fibers going between one rib and the next. The so called subcostals (Fig. 29) stretch over more than one space. Both these muscles occupy the middle two-fourths of the intercostal spaces and are especially well developed in the lower ones.

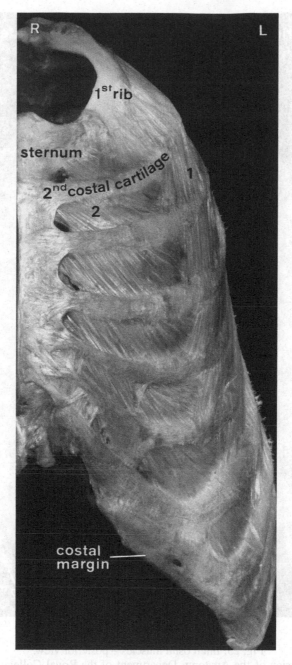

Fig. 22. Intercostal muscles – anterior view.

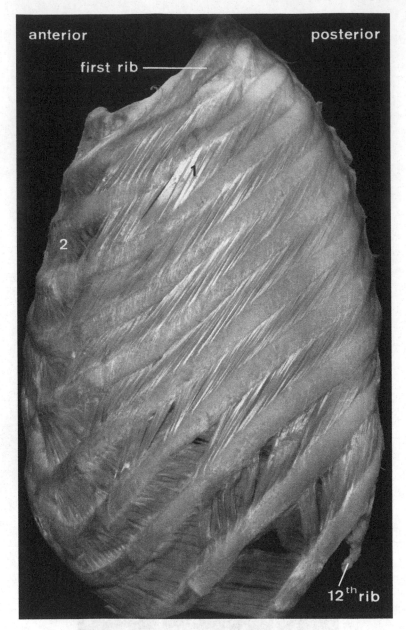

Fig. 23. Intercostal muscles – posterior view.
(By kind permission of the Anatomy Department of the Royal College of Surgeons of England.) Note: The fleshy fibers of the external layer of intercostals (1) stop close to the junction of the ribs and costal cartilages. Fibers of the internal intercostals (2) are seen through the external intercostal membrane as they arise next to the sternum.

human subjects and included the external, internal and innermost intercostals as well as two other incomplete deep muscle layers, the subcostals and sternocostalis.

Taylor demonstrated two functionally distinct layers of intercostal muscle in all parts of the chest wall. The superficial one was activated only by inspiratory efforts, and the deeper one by expiratory efforts.

In all areas of the thorax the external intercostals functioned in inspiration. (excepting of course where muscle is replaced by the external intercostal membrane). The internal intercostals functioned in expiration excepting in the parasternal regions (intercartilaginous spaces between ribs 1–4 and sometimes 5) where they also contracted in inspiration. This seemingly contradictory behaviour of the parasternal intercostals is puzzling. However, there are two layers of muscle deep to the parasternal spaces, the internal intercostals superficially and the sternocostalis, (Transversus thoracis) which functions in expiration and is deep to it.

Subsequently Campbell (1968, 1970, 1974, 1978), Sears (1973), and Basmajian (1978) confirmed and extended Taylor's studies. During voluntary (as opposed to reflex) respiration, the amount of intercostal activity may vary from limited action of the parasternal portion in quiet breathing, to alternating involvement of both layers throughout the thorax in forced respiration. *"During phonation at high lung volumes, there is contraction of the external and parasternal muscles. At low volumes, there is contraction of the internal intercostals"* (Campbell, 1974). As a result of these findings and those regarding sensory components (mechanoreceptors and sensory endings), Sears (1973, 1977) considered that the intercostals are probably more active during phonation or during voluntary maintenance of a fixed intrathoracic pressure, and since they prevent the intercostal spaces from being sucked in they can counteract the recoiling forces of the lung and chest wall. The role of the intercostals in singing will be discussed later under the heading "subglottic pressure" on pages 84-85.

c) Other muscles of inspiration

According to Campbell, Agostini and Newsom Davis (1970), and Sears (1980, un-published) the levatores costarum also aid inspiration (Fig. 24). They elevate and tend to swing the ribs outwards. Some texts also mention the serratus posterior and inferior muscles (Fig. 25), these connect the ribs to the vertebral column however they are small and thin and therefore not likely to play a powerful role at any time.

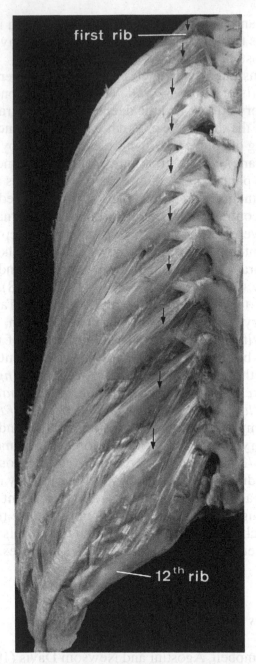

Fig. 24. Levatores costarum muscles on the posterior surface of the thorax (left side).
(By kind permission of the Anatomy Department of the Royal College of Surgeons of
England.) These small triangular muscles arise from the transverse processes of the seventh cervical and upper eleven thoracic vertebrae and are inserted between the tubercle
and angles of the rib immediately below. These muscles elevate the ribs, and because of
the length of the ribs, the anterior ends have a wide excursion.

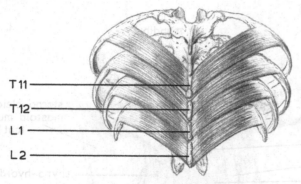

T 11

T 12

L 1

L 2

Fig. 25. Serratus posterior inferior muscles.

This muscle is paired and attached to the spines of thoracic vertebrae eleven and twelve and the first two lumbar vertebrae. It runs upwards and laterally to be attached to the lower borders of the lower three or four ribs near their angles. The serratus posterior superior (not pictured here) attaches to the spines of the seventh cervical and first three thoracic vertebrae. Despite the differing direction of the fibers, both of the serratus posterior muscles are inspiratory, the superior one raises the upper ribs and the inferior depresses the lower ribs to help stabilize them during contraction of the diaphragm.

Neck muscles like the scalenes and sternocleidomastoids are postural as well as inspiratory in function (Fig. 26). Their normal postural activity helps to stabilise and lift up the top of the rib cage whereas active contraction with the head fixed raises the rib cage. The scalenes are constantly and rhythmically active during inspiration. Overactivity of the sternocleidomastoids and muscles raising the shoulder girdle creates a type of shoulder breathing; a hinderance to good vocal production and aesthetically displeasing.

Expiration

Expiration during normal breathing or speaking is largely passive, occurring mainly by relaxation of the diaphragm, and elastic recoil of the expanded lungs and enlarged rib cage. In the erect posture gravity also will tend to drawn the ribs downwards and inwards. However, for controlled expiration during phonation, as well as for increasing the intensity or duration of sound, more muscular activity is called into play. Muscles whose actions tend to diminish the size of the thorax are considered expiratory, and there are a number capable of this.

a) The abdominal muscles

The external and internal oblique muscles and transversus abdominis are the most important and powerful muscles of expiration (Fig. 27). All

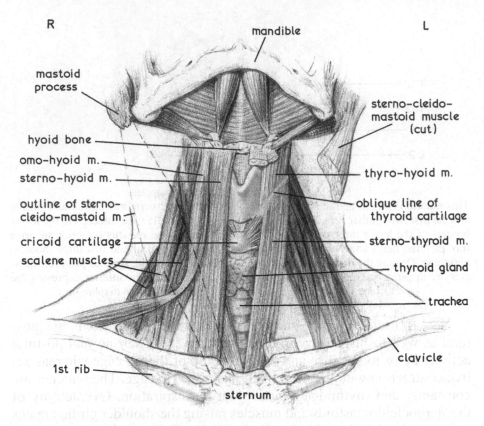

Fig. 26. Muscles of the neck.
The cut upper portion of the sternocleidomastiod muscle is shown on the left and is sche-
matically outlined on the right by the dashed lines. This paired muscle is attached to the
anterior surface of the manubrium, the medial end of the upper surface of the clavicle and
extends upwards to the mastoid process of the temporal bone and the lateral half of the
superior nuchal line.
There are three pairs of scalene muscles, the anterior, middle and posterior. Each pair arises from the transverse processes of the cervical vertebrae. Their precise upper and lower
attachments differ from each other. The anterior is inserted on the scalene tubercle on the
inner border of the first rib, the middle to the upper posterior part of the first rib, and the
posterior to the outer border of the second rib. They all assist in elevating the ribs (rather
like the lid of a box) to which they attach. They also laterally flex the neck and rotate the
cervical portion of the spinal column to the opposite side.

three pairs of these broad, flat sheets of muscle are attached to the rib
cage and parts of the iliac crest (the highest part of the pelvis). The two
deepest muscles also arise by sheet-like tendons and connective tissue
from the vertebral column and thus make a complete tube from back to
front. The external oblique reinforces the front and sides of this tube and
does not have any attachment to the spine.

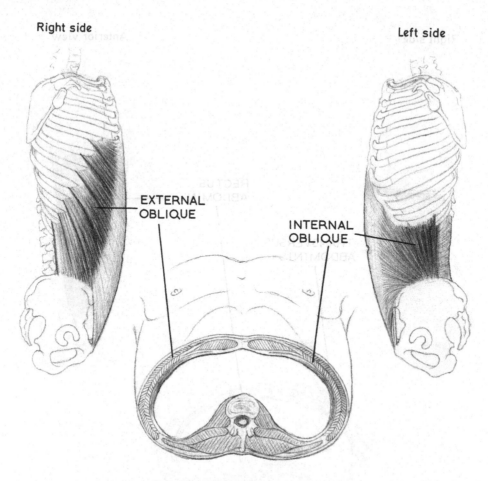

Right side

Left side

EXTERNAL
OBLIQUE

INTERNAL
OBLIQUE

Fig. 27. The external and internal oblique muscles.

The external oblique, the most superficial muscle, is attached to the outer surfaces of the lower eight ribs. The posterior fibers are attached on the outer border of the anterior two-thirds of the iliac crest and the anterior fibers slope obliquely downwards and forwards forming a sheet-like tendon (aponeurosis) which constitutes the outermost layer of the rectus sheath. The inguinal ligament, which runs between the iliac crest and the pubic tubercle is the free lower border of this muscle. This ligament forms a gutter facing upwards on the inner surface of the muscle.

The internal oblique muscle arises from the lateral portion of the inguinal ligament, the iliac crest and the lumbar fascia. The posterior fibers course upwards and are attached either as muscle or tendon to the whole of the lower border of the rib cage while the remaining fibers course forward to become tendinous and contribute to the rectus sheath.

The transversus abdominis muscle is the deepest of the three anterio-lateral abdominal muscles. It is attached to the inner surfaces of the costal cartilages of the lower six ribs (interdigitating with the diaphragm), the lumbar fascia, the iliac crest, part of the inguinal ligament and passes into a broad tendon which also contributes to the rectus sheath.

The rectus abdominis, a fourth paired muscle of the abdominal wall, extends vertically from the super-ficial portion of the fifth, sixth and seventh costal cartilages to the symphysis and upper surface of the body of the pubis. It is encased in a tough fibrous sheath formed from the aponeuroses of the three sheet-like muscles. It is obvious that it will

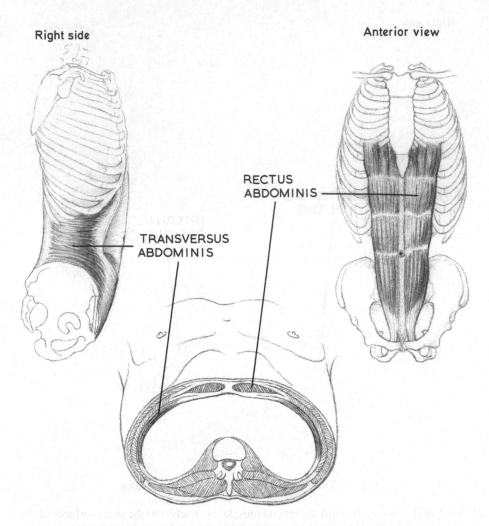

Right side

Anterior view

RECTUS
ABDOMINIS

TRANSVERSUS
ABDOMINIS

Fig. 28. The transversus abdominis and rectus abdominis muscles.

help in flexion of the spine when the trunk is raised from the supine position, however, in standing it is a most important antagonist to the post vertebral muscles of the lower spine. A pair of strap muscles, the rectus abdominis, and three pairs of flat muscles (the external and internal obliques and transversus abdominis), and their aponeuroses form a strong, flexible support for the abdominal viscera. The abdominal and pelvic cavities communicate directly with each other. From pictures of the skeleton note that the only bony supports are the vertebral column, and the pelvis formed of two hip bones, and the sacrum. The rest of the walls of the two cavities are formed of muscles and sheet-like tendons. The roof is the diaphragm, the floor is the pelvic diaphragm. The back, side and front walls are formed of the four pairs of muscles illustrated in Figs. 27 and 28. Acting together the three pairs of sheet-like muscles and their tendons raise intra-abdominal pressure and are important in forced expiration and all expulsive movement. The play an important part in rotation with flexion of the spine. Other muscles on the posterior wall of the abdomen contribute to flexion and lateral felxion of the lumbar spine. The rectus abdominis muscles are enclosed in the rectus sheath. Their actions include flexion of the lumbar vertebral column, depression of the ribs and stabilization of the pelvis during walking.

(1) All three pairs form a strong tendinous sheath around the paired, long, rectus abdominis (Fig. 28), the strap muscle on either side of the midline.
(2) All three pairs of sheet muscles acting together raise intra-abdominal pressure as in lifting, holding the breath or singing.
(3) This in turn aids upward movement of the relaxed diaphragm by pushing the abdominal organs up against it.
(4) Because of their attachment to the rib cage these sheets of muscles are important in stabilising posture and acting on the spine. Different patterns of activity can cause rotation and/or lateral bending.
(5) The rectus abdominis is a powerful flexor of the lumbar spine bal ancing the activity in the powerful post-vertebral muscles. It does not play a significant part in respiration.

Despite some references to the contrary, electromyographic studies (Campbell, 1952) show that the rectus abdominis plays little or no part in respiration, even when forced (it will act if the spine is being flexed against gravity, a movement which should not be encountered normally when singing).

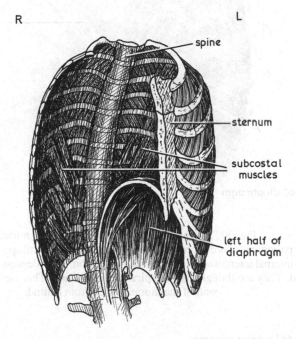

Fig. 29. Subcostal muscles. (A portion of the right side of the rib cage is cut away.) The subcostals cross more than one space and lie deep to the internal intercostal muscles in the middle two-fourths of the thoracic wall. They act with the internal intercostals in expiration (see also Fig. 21).

b) Other muscles of expiration

In addition to the important action of the abdominal muscles in expiration the internal and innermost intercostals (with the exception of the parasternal portions) and subcostals (Figs. 29 and 30) all act in expiration by diminishing the size of the thorax.

The floor of the pelvis is formed by a group of muscles, collectively called the pelvic diaphragm. It functions during singing in order to maintain abdominal balance. (These pelvic muscles act as antagonists to the diaphragm.)

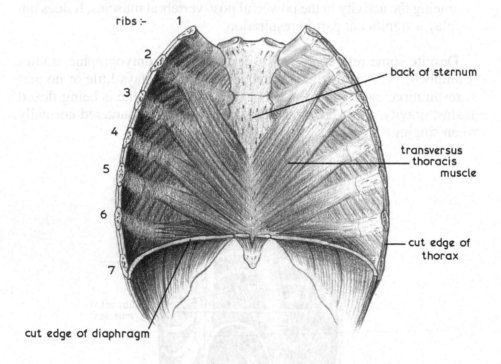

Fig. 30. Transversus thoracis (sternocostalis) muscles.
These thin, paired muscles connect the second to sixth costal cartilages to the sternum and lie deep to the internal intercostals in the parasternal region. They depress the ribs to which they are attached. They are thought to be expiratory in function. This view of the antero lateral wall of the thorax is seen from behind.

Subglottic pressure

Another importnat factor that must be considered in any discussion of expiration in relation to singing is subglottic pressure, a pressure created by the flow of expired air against partially closed (adducted) vocal folds. This is mentioned in literature relating to speech yet little attention has been given to it in relation to singing. However, teachers have long recognised the connection between subglottic pressure and vocal control because, in addition to being a factor in control of air flow, it is very important in achieving a constant intensity of sound. Abo-el-Enene (1967) and Adzaku (1980) have shown that mechanoreceptors in the subglottic mucous membrane are sensitive to changes in air pressures and exert significant reflex effects on the activity of the intrinisic muscles of the larynx. Adzaku suggests that the role of subglottic sensitivity to changes in air pressure assumes increasing importance as the air pressure rises during expiration, particularly in singing.

Dynamic balance in the vocal folds is necessarily involved in subglottic pressure and is controlled by the action of intrinsic laryngeal muscles (see Chapter 7, page 113).

Care must be taken not to confuse this tension caused by the controlled contraction of the small muscles of the larynx with bodily tension produced by contraction of the muscles of the neck. (Aspects of control of tension of the vocal folds are discussed in Chapter 7.) All too often singers try to control sound by using the neck muscles and this seriously impairs vocal function and quality.

Bouhuys (1966) has stated that phonation requires close coordination between two mechanical processes: the first determining pitch, loudness and quality of sound brought about by movements of the vocal folds and the walls of the pharynx, mouth and tongue; the second determining air-flow and subglottic pressure brought about by movements of the chest wall. To the uninitiated it might appear that air-flow is responsible for generating a tone of constant or increasing loudness. However Rubin, LeCover and Vennard (1967), and Bouhuys (1966) found that subglottic pressure is far more important in controlling intensity of sound. The ability of a singer to sustain a steady subglottic pressure or to vary it at will results from accurate voluntary control of inspiratory intercostal effort at high lung volumes, together with the use of the abdominal muscles acting across a gradually relaxing diaphragm. At first these actions supplement and they later counteract elastic forces at lower lung volumes (Proctor 1968, 1980).

In singing, subglottic pressure (Fig. 31) varies from 2 to 50 cm H_2O. The air-flow varies between 100–200 ml per second. A moderate tone has been shown to generate 10 cm H_2O of pressure and singing a very loud crescendo can generate pressures as high as 50–60 cm H_2O (Proctor, 1980). Two factors interfere with efficient maintenance of subglottic pressure and impair vocal quality by causing excessive glottal tensions.

These are uncoordinated use of the muscles of the abdominal wall and thorax, and contraction of the musculature of the vocal tract leading to disturbance of flow-pressure relationships (Rubin et al., 1967). Such changes in subglottic pressure induce reflex alterations in respiration, such as variation in rate and depth.

To generate a constant subglottic pressure for singing, a graded, coordinated action of the inspiratory and expiratory muscles is required, and physiologists, for example Sears (1977), consider the intercostal muscles ideally suited for this task. These muscles have mechanoreceptors which allow fine regulation and gradation in their actions, therefore they are capable of causing delicate adjustments in air pressure.

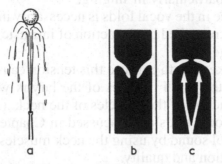

a   b   c

Fig. 31. Schematic illustration of the principle of subglottic pressure.
A constant air pressure below the vocal folds will help to maintain proper intensity of sound. The simile of "the sound sitting on a cushion of air" is often used by teachers of singing. This is pictured here as a ball balanced on a jet of water (a). In (b) with the vocal folds not fully adducted, resistance to an upward flow of air is less than in (c) where they are fully opposed.

Summary: breathing for singing

Observation, experience and physiological evidence show that patterns of breathing for singing differ from those of typical respiration. Sustaining a tone at constant air pressure and intensity, and varying the pitch for the duration of musical phrases is fundamental to the art of singing. Therefore an essential part of the singer's technique is learning to breathe efficiently for sustaining sound. This type of breathing depends of the integrated effort of the many postural, inspiratory and expiratory muscles. Sears (1977) has aptly pointed out that *"the precise pattern of activity in the individual singer will be completely idiosyncratic, depending on many factors including the basic shape of his rib cage and the manner in which he holds it when singing."*

Therefore the way in which a singer maintains the balance of his rib cage and his body, that is to say his posture and alignment, are highly significant. (All the following discussions assume that posture is correct.) Excessive tension in muscles of the jaw, mouth, tongue, pharynx, and neck, revealed by noisy breath-taking, inhibits free vibration of the vocal folds. Tension in muscles of the shoulder and chest affects the singer's estimation of how much air is needed or is available for use. A false sense of fullness can be produced which misleads the singer into believing that he has an adequate supply, and only when he begins to sing does he realise that little air was taken in and therefore very little breath is available. Abdominal muscles that are too strongly contracted act as antagonists to the diaphragm which is then prevented from contracting adequately. This is often the case with young women who have been told: "Hold in your stomach", consequently they have a difficult time relaxing the abdominal muscles during efficient inspiration.

Inhalation is most efficient when there is no effort involved. For this to be accomplished the vocal tract (oropharyngeal airway) has to be balanced and relaxed, widely open, offering a low resistance to the incoming air. For an optimum inspiration air enters through the mouth, the soft palate being elevated, tongue and oropharyngeal muscles relaxed, and the abdominal muscles slightly relaxed however not to the extent of producing an unsightly protrusion of the abdomen. When all these factors are operative the singer is able to breathe noiselessly and control the amount of air brought into the lungs.

Support of tone is dependent upon maintenance of subglottic pressure. This is done by the maintenance of postural balance, including the position of the rib cage, which in turn allows the abdominal muscles and diaphragm to function efficiently.

The balanced position of the rib cage implies a comfortable (and not fixed or rigid) chest position so that there is no interference with the vibratory mechanism and no counteraction of expiratory effort. An inexperienced singer tends to allow the rib cage to be drawn downwards by the increasing expiratory effort, and great concentration is needed to overcome this. A singer whose stance is faulty and therefore inefficient will be sorely tried by the patience needed to unlearn old habits before replacing them with new efficient ones; however the benefits justify the effort.

Singers spend a great deal of time learning how to begin a tone properly. The coordination of the onset of tone, or the "attack", is critical to phrasing and efficient use of air. At the point of attack the inspiratory muscles continue their activity and the abdominal muscles now also contract as described so well by Sears (1977):

"If the abdominal muscles are not contracted as exhalation and phonation commence, then the weight of the abdominal viscera distends

*the abdominal wall outwards and through the slack diaphragm exerts
an expiratory, collapsing force on the rib cage. The importance of the
abdominal muscle contraction… is that it supports the weight of the
viscera and, by so doing, relieves the rib cage of an appreciable gravita-
tional load. At the same time, by increasing the abdominal pressure, the
contracting abdominal wall passively tenses the diaphragm. In turn this
imposes a lifting force on the rib cage, in effect allowing it to be held by
less inspiratory muscle force …"*

The action of the abdominal and pelvic muscles, combined with
dynamic balance and alignment continued from inspiration, ensures a
steady expiratory flow of air, while the subglottic pressure regulates intensity of sound. This regulation can now occur because contraction of
the abdominal wall and resultant support of the chest helps, with the
diaphragm, to form a stable base or platform. *"Against this base below,
and the resistance to the airflow of the phonating vocal folds above, the
short, rapidly acting intercostal muscles can compress the rib cage and
lungs and thus increase subglottal pressure for the stressed segments of
speech or song"* (Sears, 1977).

The act of breathing for singing involves a dynamic interplay between postural muscles and those of respiration. There is a pattern of
movement and balance which allows the singer freedom of his instrument. A very short time (200–300 milliseconds, Wilder 1979) before the
act of singing a phrase, a pattern of coordinated activity is initiated in the
muscles of respiration to ensure proper subglottic pressure. The singer's
ability to initiate this complex process automatically can only come after
desirable patterns have been practised until they have become habitual
and unconscious. A well-trained singer will have a pre-formed mental
concept for each phrase or song, and proper management of breathing
will become spontaneous. This is accomplished by trial, error and performing experience. Once this process is acquired and programmed the
artist can take command of the act of singing. He can only develop fully
as an artist when the muscular control has become an unconscious reflex
and his concentration is devoted to interpretation. As Winckel (1967) has
stated so beautifully: *"… breath is the liaison between the excitement of
feeling and the physiological effects. The trained singer especially feels
this, since he must form the tone on the breath as a modulating process
– and his success – apart from the mastering of the basic technique – is
qualitatively dependent upon requirements in the area of the soul."*

Phonation 7

Of all the animals capable of voicing recognisable noises and signals, only man is capable of articulation and communication in words. Too often this ability to vocalise is taken for granted and the vulnerability of the vocal mechanism is ignored until it is spoiled by misuse. It is hoped that the discussion of the structure and function of the larynx will increase the understanding of teachers, therapists and students and will encourage exploration of the options they have in keeping the mechanism healthy.

As mentioned previously, all sound-producing parts of the body have at least one other function and the larynx is no exception. While sound production is an important function of the larynx, its primary function is to act as a protective valve at the top of the trachea (wind pipe) preventing foreign material from entering the lower air passages and lungs. In addition to protecting the lungs, this valve closes tightly in order to help to sustain pressure in the thorax and abdomen when one lifts heavy objects or strains as in parturition, micturition or defecation. In swallowing, the breath is automatically held and the vocal folds close tightly, thus preventing food from entering the lower respiratory passages. Anyone who has had food go down "the wrong way" will appreciate the sensitivity of this protective function of the larynx and throat. When particles larger than 3/1000 of a millimeter pass through the vocal folds, a powerful cough reflex is initiated.

Muscles are utilised in singing and, like those in the rest of the body, they are subject to fatigue, disease and emotional factors. Failure to realise this and take appropriate rest periods can lead to vocal abuse that may jeopardise a singer's career. Because the vibratory mechanism includes muscles, it is important to warm up as athletes do before a practice or performance. Improper or insufficient vocal warm-up is a potent cause of vocal fatigue and inefficiency.

The anatomy of the vibratory mechanism

The larynx is a simple-looking structure, and this belies the subtlety and complexity of its function. It has a skeleton of cartilages with joints; its joints are held by ligaments and operated by small muscles (Figs. 32 and 33). It is connected above by a common air and food passage, and below communicates directly with the trachea. Ordinary movements of the head, neck and those of respiration mean that the larynx and trachea must also be mobile. Thus, the larynx is suspended and supported from in front and behind, and above and below by paired muscles. It is slung from above, in front and behind through the intermediacy of the hyoid bone.

The mobility of the larynx can be easily ascertained by placing a finger on the laryngeal prominence (Adam's apple) and swallowing; it will rise on swallowing and will descend as one takes a deep breath. These movements are due to the contraction or relaxation of the various muscle attachments and the elasticity of the trachea, bronchial trees and lungs.

When the larynx is built up gradually by beginning inferiorly, it will be easier to visualise. The foundation is the cricoid cartilage which is shaped like a signet ring with the signet facing backwards, or posteriorly (Fig. 34). Its lumen leads directly to the trachea. It is attached to the thyroid cartilage by means of a pair of joints (the crico-thyroid articulation) and by ligaments and muscles.

On the upper border of the posterior portion of the cricoid are two small pyramidal-shaped cartilages called the arytenoids, the details of which are shown in Figs. 34 and 35B. These are connected to the cricoid by means of ligaments and muscles and are capable of complex movements. The crico-arytenoid joint surfaces are subtly shaped to allow for rotation as well as gliding motions. Anything attached to the front will pull them downwards; anything attached to the top or the peak will pull them backwards. These movements are caused by the muscles that attach to the muscular processes (sides) and the muscles and ligaments attaching to the vocal processes (front).

The thyroid cartilage is shaped like a shield and is concave posteriorly (Fig. 35A, 35B, 35C). Its anterior prominence is the protrusion in the neck recognised as the "Adam's apple" (most obvious in late adolescence or maturity, and more so in males than females).

The thyroid, cricoid and lower portions of the arytenoid cartilages are composed of a type of cartilage known as hyaline which can calcify and even ossify (become bone) thus losing elasticity as a person ages. In addition, the lubricating joint fluid becomes more viscous (thicker) with age and affects the ease of movements of the joints. Therefore, the

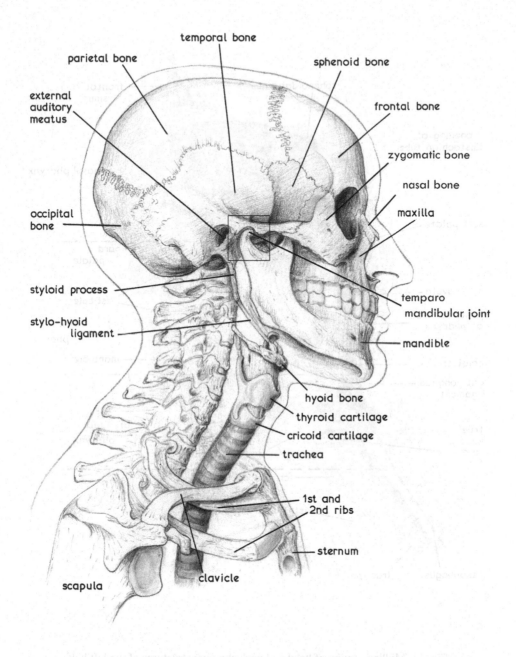

Fig. 32. Skeleton of the head and neck (right side).
Note: The cartilages of the larynx have no articulations with any of these structures. The stylo-hyoid ligament, which is illustrated here, and muscles from the mandible, skull, pharynx, soft palate, tongue, hyoid and strap muscles are the structures that maintain the position of the larynx. Details of these slings and supports are given in Chapter V (see also Fig. 51).

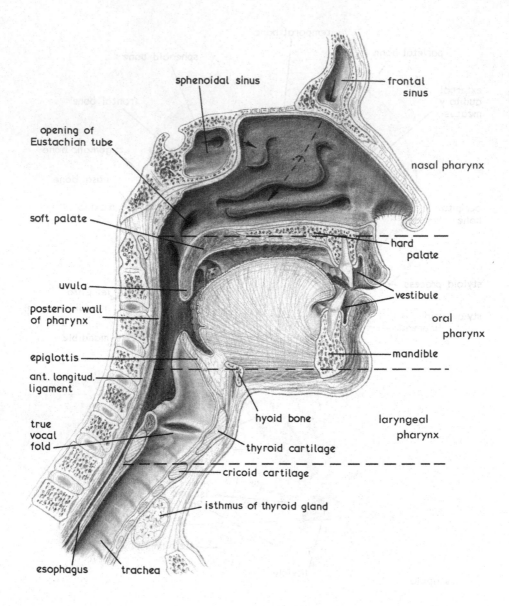

Fig. 33. Midline section of head and neck showing structures of the left half.
Note: *1*. The communication of the nose and mouth with the pharynx. *2*. The crossing of the
pathways for air and food. *3*. The extensive area of tongue facing the pharynx and normally
invisible from the mouth.

age at which these changes occur can have a direct bearing on a singer's muscular responsiveness, quality of voice and vocal agility in florid passages. It is difficult to state the exact age as which these changes begin; X-rays reveal highly variable findings. Ossification can begin at any time after puberty, and may be delayed until the middle sixties. For example, X-rays of two singers aged 32 showed that one had almost complete ossification of all the laryngeal cartilages and the other had none (Bunch, 1976).

The epiglottis is an elastic cartilage which is attached to the thyroid cartilage by means of a ligament, and it looks like a curled leaf (Fig. 35B). During swallowing it folds over to cover the entrance to the larynx. It is partly pulled down by the small muscles underlying the aryepiglottic folds (Fig. 36b) and partly pushed by the back of the tongue as the action of swallowing pulls the larynx up and forward. This movement of the epiglottis combined with the strong closure of the vocal folds prevents food from entering the air passages.

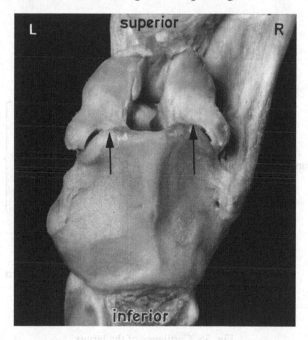

Fig. 34. Crico-arytenoid articulations seen from behind.
(By kind permission of the Anatomy Department of the Royal College of Surgeons of England.) The paired synovial crico-arytenoid articulations (↑) allow: (*1*) a rotational movement of the arytenoids which moves the vocal process laterally or medially; (2) a gliding movement which permits the arytenoid cartilages to move towards or away from each other.
Because of the shape of the articular facets, the movements of gliding and rotation are concomitant. Medial gliding occurs with medial rotation (adduction of the vocal folds), and lateral gliding with lateral rotation (abduction of the vocal folds).

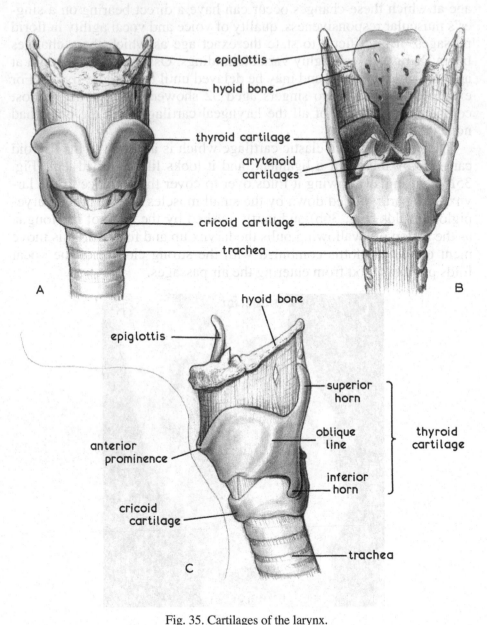

Fig. 35. Cartilages of the larynx.
Note: The inferior cornu (horn) of the thyroid articulates with the cricoid cartilage. This synovial joint permits a forward or backward rocking movement.

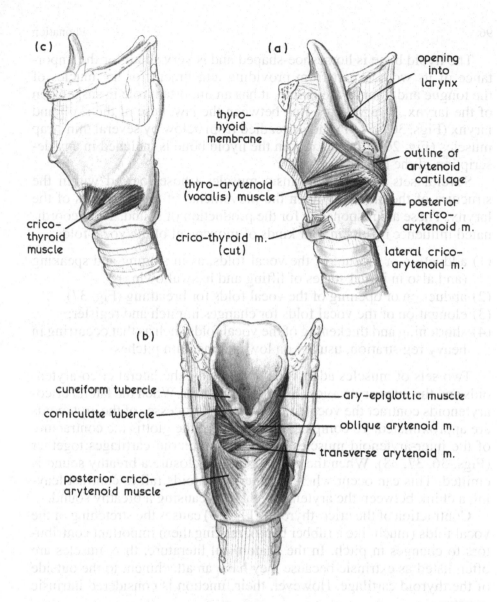

Fig. 36. Intrinsic muscles of the larynx.

The paired *lateral crico-arytenoids (a)* are attached to the lateral and superior portions of the cricoid cartilage, and the tips of the vocal processes of the arytenoid cartilages.

The *interarytenoid (b)* muscle is attached to the posterior surface of both arytenoid cartilages.

The *crico-thyroid (c)* muscle is paired and attached to the anterior portion of the cricoid cartilage and the inferior horn and inner and outer edges of the lower border of the thyroid cartilage.

The paired *thyro-arytenoid (a)* muscle consists of two parts: the *internal thyro-arytenoid* or *vocalis* which forms the body of the vocal fold, and the *external thyro-arytenoid* which is lateral to the vocal fold and the vestibular fold (often some of its fibers are found in the vestibular fold).

The *posterior crico-arytenoid (b)* is paired, and attached to the posterior portion of the cricoid lamina and the posterior surface of the muscular process of each arytenoid.

The hyoid bone is horseshoe-shaped and is very small for the importance of its work. Apart from providing attachment for the mucles of the tongue and floor of the mouth, it has an important role in suspension of the larynx. It serves as a link between the jaw, base of the skull and larynx (Figs. 36, 48, 51) and is steadied from below by several thin strap muscles (Fig. 26). For this reason the hyoid bone is included in any description of the larynx.

Several sets of paired intrinsic muscles (those located within the structure of the larynx) govern the movements of the cartilages of the larynx. These are responsible for the production of sound. Their coordinated influence results in four kinds of movement of the vocal folds:

(1) adduction or closure of the vocal folds, as in singing and speaking (and also in initial stages of lifting and in swallowing)
(2) abduction or opening of the vocal folds for breathing (Fig. 37)
(3) elongation of the vocal folds for changes in pitch and register;
(4) shortening and thickening of the vocal folds such as that occurring in heavy registration, usually on low and medium pitches.

Two sets of muscles adduct the vocal folds: the lateral crico-arytenoids and the inter-arytenoids (Figs. 36a and 36b). When the lateral crico-arytenoids contract the vocal folds and vocal processes of the arytenoids are approximated. To complete the closure of the glottis the contracture of the inter-arytenoid muscles brings the arytenoid cartilages together (Figs. 36, 37, 38). When there is incomplete closure a breathy sound is emitted. This can occur when the inter-arytenoids fail to contract leaving a chink between the arytenoids, thereby causing a breathy sound.

Contraction of the crico-thyroids (Fig. 39) causes the stretching of the vocal folds (much like a rubber band), making them important contributors to changes in pitch. In the anatomical literature, thse muscles are often listed as extrinsic because they have an attachment to the outside of the thyroid cartilage. However, their function is considered intrinsic in nature.

When the posterior crico-arytenoid muscles (Figs. 36b and 38) contract, they open the glottis by abducting the vocal folds. Therefore these muscles are phasically active throughout life during breathing. They act as antagonists to the vocalis and crico-thyroids and therefore are also involved in pitch.

The last intrinsic muscle to be discussed is the vocalis or internal thyro-arytenoid (Figs. 36a, 40, 41). It is paired and forms the main body of the vocal fold. Its contraction shortens the distance between the thyroid and arytenoids and increases the tension of the muscle. In addition, it has some ability to adduct the vocal folds.

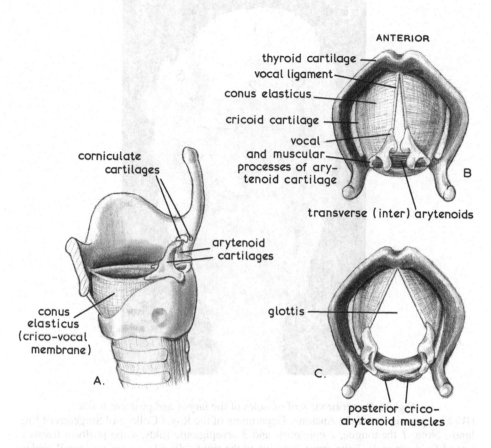

ANTERIOR

thyroid cartilage

vocal ligament

conus elasticus

cricoid cartilage

vocal
and muscular
processes of ary-
tenoid cartilage

B

corniculate
cartilages

transverse (inter) arytenoids

arytenoid
cartilages

conus
elasticus
(crico-vocal
membrane)

glottis

A.

C.

posterior crico-
arytenoid muscles

Fig. 37. Movements of the vocal folds.
Movements of the vocal folds permitted by the shape of the articular surfaces of the crico-
arytenoid joints are brought about by the muscles attached to the arytenoid cartilages.
1 The posterior crico-arytenoid muscles are the only ones capable of abducting the vocal
folds.
2 The lateral crico-arytenoid muscles cause adduction of the vocal folds.
3 The transverse and oblique interarytenoid muscles pull the arytenoids towards each other
so that their medial surfaces touch and block off the triangular opening that remains when
the vocal processes and therefore, folds are apposed.
4 The crico-thyroids are the intrinsic muscles responsible for elongating the vocal folds (see
Fig. 26 for strap muscles which assist crico-thyroid muscles).

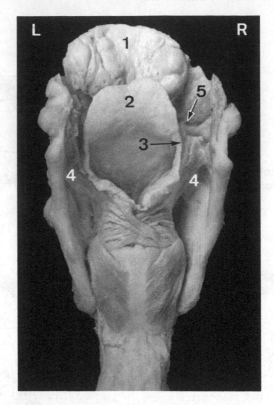

Fig. 38. Posterior view of muscles of the larynx and piriform fossae.
(By kind permission of the Anatomy Department of the Royal College of Surgeons of England.) Note: *1* the tongue, *2* epiglottis, and *3* aryepiglottic folds, *4* the piriform fossae or lateral food channels, *5* the arrow pointing to the right vellecula, one of two small pockets behind the tongue into which fluids collect and then overflow into the lateral food channels.

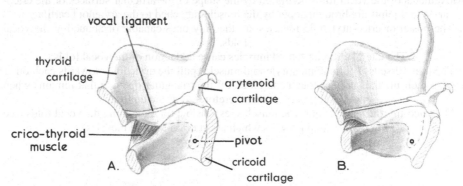

Fig. 39. Action of the crico-thyroid muscles.
The crico-thyroid muscles pull the thyroid cartilage torward and tilt the cricoid cartilage backward, thus elongating the vocal ligaments and increasing tension. The figure on the left *(A)* shows the vocal ligaments slack with no contraction of the crico-thyroids, and on the right *(B)* the tension and elongation are evident.

There are two sets of folds in the larynx: the true vocal folds and the false folds (vestibular) (Figs. 40 and 41). The true vocal folds are made up of the vocalis muscle, the vocal processes of the arytenoid cartilages, and the vocal ligament which is the free upper edge of a thickened membrane called the conus elasticus which arises from the upper surface of the cricoid cartilage (Fig. 37a). The conus elasticus is a strong supporting structure of the vocalis muscle and the vocal fold. The false or vestibular folds consist mostly of fatty tissue, and of mucous glands which help lubricate the true folds. There are some pathological conditions in which sound may be made by the vestibular folds but normally they are retracted during phonation and do not contribute to sound. However, they are important because they are involved in lubrication of the vocal folds and thereby prevent frictional damage during phonation.

Between the vocal folds and vestibular folds lies a tiny saccule or ventricle (Fig. 40). This saccule is lined with mucous glands, the primary

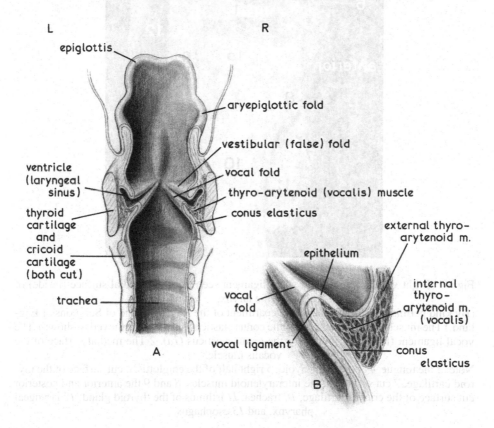

Fig. 40. Folds of the larynx.
A is a coronal section through the larynx and trachea, *B* a more detailed coronal section of the right vocal fold.

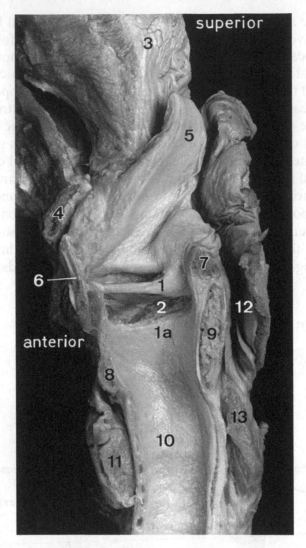

Fig. 41. Right vocalis muscle and vocal ligament seen from the medial surface (inside) of the larynx.
(By kind permission of the Anatomy Department of the Royal College of Surgeons of England.) The muscles and greater part of the conus elasticus have been removed to show: *1* The vocal ligament (free upper border of the conus elasticus *(1a)*. *2* The medial surface of the vocalis muscle.
Note: *3* the tongue, *4* body of the hyoid, *5* right half of the epiglottis, *6* cut surface of the thyroid cartilage, *7* cut surface of the interarytenoid muscles, *8* and *9* the anterior and posterior cut surface of the cricoid cartilage, *10* trachea, *11* isthmus of the thyroid gland, *12* laryngeal pharynx, and *13* esophagus.

function of which in man is laryngeal lubrication. The presence of the ventricle permits free, unimpeded movements of the vocal folds and perhaps acts as an acoustic filter to reduce some of the higher harmonic

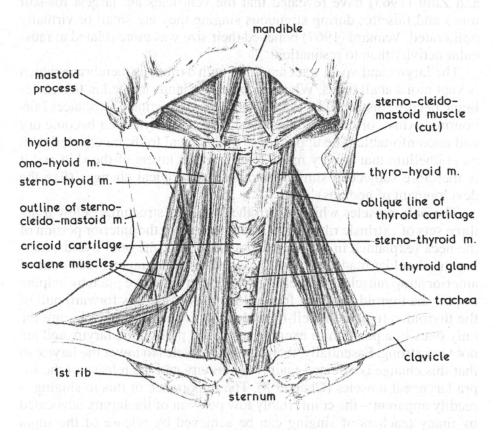

Fig. 42. Anterior view of dissection of the strap muscles, part of the contractile mechanism for supporting and depressing the larynx.

NB: The sterno-hyoid of the right side has been pulled laterally and the left one has been removed. Normally the medial borders of these muscles touch.

The *omo-hyoid* arises from the scapula and is attached to the hyoid bone, thus acting as a guy rope from below and posteriorly.

The *thyro-hyoid* is attached to the oblique line of the thyroid cartilage and to the hyoid bone.

The *sterno-hyoid* arises from the superior part of the sternum and is attached to the hyoid bone, forming a guy rope from below and anteriorly.

The *sterno-thyroid* is attached to the superior part of the sternum and to the oblique line of the thyroid cartilage, forming another tie from below and anteriorly.

Note: these muscles are counterbalanced by ones arising from above the larynx; only the digastric and mylo-hyoid can be seen in this view (see Fig. 48 for details of muscles suspending and acting upon the larynx as a whole).

vibrations above the glottis which tend to make the voice harsh (Kirchner, 1970). Some studies have linked these ventricles with resonation. Special X-ray (tomograph) studies by van den Berg (1955) and Landeau and Zuili (1963) have revealed that the ventricles are largest for soft tones and falsetto; during strenuous singing they are small or virtually obliterated. Vennard (1967) believed their size was more related to muscular activity than to resonation.

The larynx and vocal tract are lined with a mucous membrane which is kept moist at all times. When the mucous glands located in this membrane become disturbed by infections or disease, irritant substances (airbourne toxins), or emotion, the vocal tract and larynx can become dry and uncomfortable. The upper edges of the vocal folds are covered with an epithelium that is very much like the outer layers of the skin and it is therefore subject to similar kinds of pathological changes (like the development of nodules).

The only muscles which attach the larynx to structures below it are three sets of extrinsic ribbon-like strap muscles in the anterior portion of the neck (explained in Fig. 42), and another pair, the omo-hyoids, uniting the shoulder blade and hyoid. According to Sonninen (1956) one of anterior strap muscles, the sterno-thyroid, can influence pitch by helping to pull the thyroid cartilage forward. He has noted this forward pull of the thyroid cartilage on well-trained singers. The strap muscles are the only ones in a position to exert a downward pull on the larynx and are not very strong. Essentially, there are few muscles to lower the larynx so that this change is effected mainly by gravity and the release of the supra laryngeal muscles (Chapter 8). The importance of this to singing is readily apparent – the comfortably low position of the larynx advocated by many teachers of singing can be achieved by release of the supra laryngeal musculature balanced by strap muscle activity and gravity.

The function of the vocal folds in singing

The commonly accepted theory of the mechanism of phonation is the myoelastic-aerodynamic theory (van den Berg, 1966). The interpretation of this theory is as follows: just before a singer's first note is sounded the vocal folds begin to close; the breath then streams from the lungs and pushes against the partially adducted (or closed) folds, initiating vibratory activity that allows puffs of air to escape and sound to be produced. This myoelastic-aerodynamic theory is based on two observations: first, that the vocal folds are adducted in response to nerve impulses transmitted from the brain to the muscles of the larynx; and second, that the process of making a sound is completed when air moves from the lungs and confined space of the trachea and subglottic area through the glottis to a larger space, thus causing a fall of pressure immediately above the level of the vocal folds which are then sucked or drawn together (the Bernoulli principle). Both the neuromuscular and aerodynamic factors must be present for phonation because the vibration of the vocal folds is not self-activating (for review, see Vennard, 1967). This motion of the vocal folds during singing involves oscillating movements that vary with the sound produced (see registration, pages 109–113).

The onset of sound

It is important to good singing to know how the vocal folds close at the onset of sound – that is, how accurately and precisely they meet in the midline. The attack involves a precise coordination of the onset of sound, the oscillating movement and the opening and closing of the folds. The ideal attack is one in which the breath begins to flow gently and is followed by a precise momentary closure of the vocal folds which meets this stream of air. When correctly done, this attack is crisp, clear and without tension. The exact terminology relating to the attack is confusing. Garcia (1894) referred to it as the "coup de glotte"; Vennard (1967) has called it the "imaginary aspirate". Garcia confounded the issue by using the term "plosive" which now, in some circles, is used to refer to the incorrect, hard glottal attack which sounds like a click. Since Garcia, the terms "coup de glotte", "glottal plosive" and "glottal stroke" have become muddled in the literature. However, an acceptable term to use is "coup de glotte" or, better still, "stroke of the glottis" because it denotes a gentle, precise touching of the vocal folds at the onset of sound.

There are two extremes of attack that are detrimental to artistic singing and ultimately to the health of the vocal folds. The first is termed "glottal plosive", (called by many other names including "hard attack" and "glottal shock" or "stop")which occurs when the vocal folds close completely before the beginning of phonation and air pressure from the lungs builds up beneath the folds causing them to burst open with an audible click at the onset of sound. Henderson (1920) has described this kind of singing as hens clucking on stage. This occurs when a singer takes a breath and then holds it, the vocal folds close tightly to hold the breath and when the tone is begun the folds burst apart literally causing a minor explosion – the glottal plosive. Winckel (1967) has described this acoustically as follows:

"Let us remember that an extremely harsh sound attack which is equivalent to a switching transient[1] emits a very broad and close fre-

quency spectrum (page 129) and therefore gives a noisy impression, that of a click. The noisiness of a sudden onset of a sound can be heard very clearly when one intones a vowel with a hard glottal stop. As opposed to this, a soft, pressureless, swelling vowel sound begins noiselessly. In the case of the hard attack, we have a situation involving physical transients, not simply a mechanical noise of the opening and closing of the vocal folds."

In addition to producing an unpleasant sound, the vocal folds are harmed by a hard attack because it is a violent motion which creates a large amount of friction between the vibrating folds similar to that occurring when coughing or clearing the throat.

The second extreme of attack is the breathy one caused by failure to coordinate air flow and closure of the vocal folds. Either the air flow is too fast and/or under so much pressure that it prevents the vocal folds from coming together properly, or muscles, for example the inter-arytenoids, are inefficient causing loss of air through the resultant chink (Fig. 37). This breathy sound is characteristic of whispering, when the vocal folds are closed yet the chink between the vocal processes of the arytenoids remains open.

Coordinating air flow with the onset of sound is difficult for the beginner who must also think of rhythm, pitch and quality of voice. However voice teachers know, and singers soon learn, that before a sound is made there must be a clear concept of the desired one. In well-coordinated singing, the vocal muscular system is pre-tuned in response to this mental concept several milliseconds before phonation. A singer who begins to utter a sound without prior thought will encounter many problems such as scooping or entering under pitch, articulating off the beat, and undesirable tension of the muscles of the larynx. As Winckel (1976) has stated:

"We can observe extremely varied attacks in the human voice. Deficient physiological preparedness (which may include a lack of mental concentration) while singing prevents the resonant areas of the physiological system from vibrating completely at the very beginning. Only after the vocal cords have begun to vibrate does the thus unprepared singer correct the adjustment of the inner resonant cavities until the optimal resonance is achieved. The aesthetic effect is unsatisfactory if the head tone with high overtones begins alone and the chest tone then follows, while the reverse is equally unsatisfactory. When the attack is correct, that is, when the inner adjustment is correct, a colourful healthy tone,

---

[1] A transient is a momentary change in sound, often noise.

which can develop naturally from piano *is immediately in evidence. Corrections made after the attack cause inconsistencies in the 'ideal' condition, which means one approaching an exponential function, and are perceived as adjustments and therefore as sound distortions."*

Neurological factors of phonation

Electromyographic studies by Faaborg-Andersen (1965), Hirano et al. (1970), Wyke (1967, 1969), and Wyke and Kirchner (1974) have shown that just prior to each phonemic[2] utterance, motor unit activity is increased in all the adductor muscles of the vocal folds. Aerodynamic research by Bouhuys et al. (1966, 1968), Ladefoged (1974), Wyke (1974), and others has shown that prior to each phonemic utterance, expiratory air flow begins and pressure below the glottis begins to rise. Wyke has suggested that this early muscular activity constitutes voluntary prephonatory tuning.

Wyke (1976) has described phonation as having three control systems. The first is the voluntary prephonatory tuning performed by the intrinsic muscles of the larynx, the intercostal muscles and the abdominal muscles. The second is the reflex modulation of this tuning during phonation which is mediated by the activity of receptor nerve endings (mechanoreceptors, page 27) in the intrinsic laryngeal muscles, the subglottic mucosa (mucous membrane), and the capsules of the laryngeal joints (crico-thyroid and crico-arytenoid). The third control is provided by acoustic auto-monitoring which is probably of particular importance to singers early in their training and work but is of less value to the seasoned performer. The well-trained singer develops a kind of awareness of sound which comes from factors of sensation in the vocal tract, vibrations of the bones of the head and the mouth and face (see discussion of oro-facial feedback in Leandersen, 1972). This awareness of sound by feel rather than by auditory feedback enables the singer to sing under almost any circumstances. A highly damped or dead concert hall can be a discouraging factor in any peformance (and even contribute to stage fright) however, proper training can help minimise the student's need for auditory feedback.

Physiological factors of phonation

Vennard (1967) has outlined five physiological factors in laryngeal function: (1) motor power produced by the flow of air (chapter 3);

---

[2] A phoneme is the smallest unit of speech sound, in some cases a syllable.

(2) contraction of the lateral crico-arytenoids and (3) contraction of the interarytenoid muscles the two factors necessary for complete adduction of the vocal folds, by him named medial compression; (4) pitch, which depends on the longitudinal stretch and the thickness of the vocal folds; and (5) registration, which comes from the relative activity or passivity of the vocalis muscles in the vocal folds. The first three factors already have been discussed. However, pitch, registration and the related topics of range, vibrato and subglottic pressure are complex and, while they are somewhat inter-related, they will be discussed separately for the sake of clarity.

Pitch

The pitch of the human voice is determined by the frequency with which the vocal folds vibrate. That is, if the singer is singing the pitch A440 then the vocal folds are vibrating, or opening and closing, 440 times per second. A higher pitch, or increased frequency, occurs when the vocal fold is lengthened and therefore made thinner and the vocalis muscle is stretched by the contraction of the crico-thyroid muscles (Fig. 39). The greater the length of the vocal folds, the higher the pitch, until at the maximum contraction point of the crico-thyroids, only the stretched vocal ligaments are vibrating. At that point, still higher pitches can be obtained by increased air flow or by a further shortening of the vocalis by its own contraction which creates damping where only part of the folds vibrate. Pitch is thought to be aided by the contraction of the sterno-thyroids (Fig. 42) (Sonninen, 1968) and by the action of the posterior crico-arytenoids acting as antagonists to the crico-thyroids (Zemlin, 1997). To lower the pitch, the tension on the crico-thyroids is decreased, thereby allowing the vocal folds to become thicker.

The singer is often vulnerable to criticism regarding his pitch. Pitch to the singer is a perception of tone-colour rather than a mathematical entity. As pointed out by Winckel (1967), Schönberg (1922) supports this concept by saying:

"I cannot accept the distinction between tone colour and pitch as it is generally stated. I find that tone makes itself noticed through colour, one dimension of which is pitch. Tone colour is the large area, of which pitch is one division."

In fact, some of the most off-pitch singing is done by those persons with "perfect pitch" who try to make the pitch by tensing parts of the vocal tract. The result is distortion of the resonating chamber of the vocal tract and consequent damping of desirable features of sound; thus, they are off-pitch (Fig. 43). Winckel (1967) emphasizes this by stating: *"A tone rich in overtones has a greater stability against pitch fluctuation than one poor in overtones. Inner modulation of sound is particularly variable in the human voice."* He further suggests that electroacoustical instruments have been able to attain greater accuracy in presentation of note values with the surprising result that the idealised tones are dull and unexciting. The question then arises *"Is a certain inaccuracy in intonation actually necessary for a satisfying auditory impression?"* It would appear to be so from perception studies on pitch and vibrato (see page). However, this does not relieve the singer of the responsibility of producing correct pitches and of being 'in tune'.

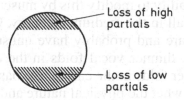

Fig. 43. Schematic representation ot the concept ot pitch.
As stated in the text, pitch for the singer includes a number of variables including hearing, registration and resonance factors, and muscular tensions which can cause pitch to alter. Here pitch is depicted as a ball with shadings that represent possible ways of alteration. Tensions which effect damping of high partials can cause the tone to sound flat, even if the pitch is correctly perceived by the singer. Likewise, the tensions which effect damping of low partials make a tone sound sharp.

Range

The artistically acceptable range for most singers is two to two-and-a-half octaves although they can produce notes of higher and lower pitch. Singers with a range of from four to five octaves are exceptional. A voice teacher aims to help the singer develop his or her range to the utmost so that the performing pitches are secure and of good quality A singer cannot expect to be able to sing in public the highest or lowest note of which he is capable. It is a common misconception that singers are given various classifications such as soprano, mezzo-soprano and contralto in terms of their range of pitches. Singers in all three of these classifications will have almost identical ranges and with training all will be able to sing a high C. However, the quality of that high C will most likely be better when the soprano sings it. Classification of voices is made chiefly according to where the best quality of tone is located in the voice, and where the depth and ease of sound are located within the range of pitches.

Cleveland (1976) has found that the quality of the speaking voice is often an indication of the correct classification for a singing voice. The higher part of the range is of better quality for the soprano, the middle for the mezzo, and low-middle for the contralto. It is a serious mistake to classify a beginner on the basis of a limited range. As the singer's training progresses and vocal freedom ensues the range expands and the area of true quality emerges.

Physiologically, the maximum range of pitch is determined by the length and shape of the singer's vocal folds and ability to coordinate the vocal muscles with the rest of the body. The quality, as distinct from pitch, of the voice is, in part, determined by the inherent shape of the vocal tract and the ability to modify this by muscular activity (see Chapter 5). Most voices fall in the medium category. Coloratura sopranos or bassi profundi are rare and probably have unusual structures (such as congenitally shorter, thinner vocal folds in the case of the coloratura, and the thicker, longer folds in the case of the basso). A good laryngologist can tell a singer what the physical nature and structure of his larynx is like, however not how well he can sing.

Vibrato

The artistic quality of singing is frequently judged by the presence of vibrato in the sound. Seashore (1938) has defined a good vibrato as a "pulsation of pitch usually accompanied with synchronous pulsations of loudness and timbre, of such extent and rate as to give a pleasing flexibility, tenderness and richness to the tone". Ideally, vibrato occurs in practically all tones of artistic singing (unless deliberately left out), and is also present in sustained tones of various instruments. A good singer will have an average vibrato of from five to eight regular pulsations per second (see studies by Seashore (1938), Vennard (1971), Large (1971), Shipp and Izdebski (1975), Shipp, Leandersen and Sundberg (1981), and Hirano (1985). Pulsations slower than five per second are easily picked up by the human ear as separate pitches, and are unpleasant. This excessively slow vibrato is often referred to as a wobble and can be caused by muscle fatigue, emotional tension or excessive contraction of the intrinsic muscles of the larynx (Sonninen, 1970; Sonninen and Damsté, 1972). A rate of much more than eight pulsations per second is normally too fast and produces either an unpleasant sound like a bleat or tremolo³, and is often caused by too much pressure on the vocal folds.

Because the vibrato creates the *illusion* of true pitch, a listener can tolerate a deviation from true pitch as large as a semitone. A good vibrato has regular intervals and rate and is consistent around the pitch. Rigidly true intonation without any vibrato would be uninteresting and intolerable (Seashore (1938), Winckel (1967)).

The influence of today's rock, pop and discotheque music has taken its toll of the vibrato. Many of these groups adhere to a singing style that resembles yelling or shouting, and the utterance of straight "white" sounds; and this kind of singing tends to iron out the vibrato and puts an enormous strain on the vocal apparatus. The strain is obvious when one sees the shear physical effort needed to produce the sound (evidenced by the large number of neck muscles that are visible when these people sing). As a result of this influence, the young student today often has difficulty in accepting a vocal sound which includes vibrato and may even reject it as sounding too "operatic".

Considerable acoustic research has been directed toward vibrato, yet virtually nothing is known about the physiological mechanism that produces it; and no one has yet explained why vibrato pulsations are sometimes seen in singers' necks in the area of the larynx. These are not to be confused with rapid movements of the jaw, the result of faulty technique. In 1925, Schilling suggested that vibrato was caused by oscillations of subglottic pressure. Since then, the more widely held view is that vibrato is caused by fluctuating activity in vocal muscles (Winckel (1967, 1974), Hirano (1978)). Large (1979) suggests physiological control of vocal vibrato is a combined laryngeal and respiratory mechanism, with the laryngeal factor predominating.

Registers

The vocal folds vibrate differently at low and high pitches (Fig. 44). The different modes of vibration at these pitch levels contribute to distinct vocal qualities which singers and teachers of singing call registers. While scientists tend to approach the study of vocal registers as mechanical problems, and voice scientists as an acoustical study, singers are concerned whether the sound is of equal quality and intensity throughout the entire range of pitches. One of the finest descriptions of registers is an early one by Nadoleqzny (1923):

---

[3] Tremolo is defined by Winckel (1967) as a vibrato that is too fast and is heard as a group of tones rather than the usual single one.

"The concept of register is understood to be a series of consecutive, similar vocal tines which the musically trained can differentiate at specific places from another adjoining series of likewise internally similar tones. Its homogenous sound depends on a definite, invariable behaviour of the harmonics. These rows of tones correspond to definite objectively and subjectively perceptible vibration regions on the head, neck, and chest. The position of the larynx changes more in a natural singer during the transition from one series of tones to another than in a well trained singer. The registers are caused by a definite mechanism (belonging to that register) of tone production (vocal fold vibration, glottal shape, air consumption), which allows for a gradual transition however from one into an adjoining register. A number of these tones can actually be produced in two overlapping registers but not always with the same intensity."

These registers have been named by singers according to the subjective sensations they produce. The low register is referred to as "chest", because singing in that register produces a feeling of vibration in the upper chest and lower neck. The upper register is called "head" (female) or "falsetto" (male), because vibrations are sensed high in the head. The middle register is often called "mixed" because it has both the high and low qualities in it. This labelling of registers according to location of sensation in the body has caused considerable confusion in usage of terminology by singers, speech pathologists and physiologists. To compound the confusion, there has been relatively little agreement about the number of possible registers in the singing voice. The subject of registers is discussed in virtually every book on vocal pedagogy and in many papers on speech therapy. Much energy has been spent describing the exact pitches on which the changes of register occur. This discussion will remain dedicated to describing what physical factors are known and understood while admitting there is much more to researched and learned about the subject.

The existence of registers has been argued over the years, and research of van den Berg (1968), Vennard (1972), Large (1968,1972,1973) and Hollien et al. (1969, 1971) has put this beyond dispute. Literature in the speech sciences) describes three basic registers: the glottal fry (or a gentle popping sound made by the vocal folds on a low pitch); a large area of regular or modal voice (including middle and head registers); and falsetto and the flute and whistle registers at the extreme top. Glottal fry is not used in song, however some teachers use it as a way to release tension in the vocal folds. Perhaps the real question is whether registration is purely a function of the vocal folds or a combination of factors including the supra-glottic vocal tract. As yet, there are no satisfactory answers to this problem.

Van den Berg and Vennard made a film (this film is still one of the finest examples of laryngeal anatomy), *The Vibrating Larynx* (1953), which shows the action of the vocal folds in low and high registers in a trained and an untrained singer and in excised larynges. The abrupt changes in the vibrational patterns of the vocal folds as they adjust from low, or heavy registration, pitches to high, or light registration, pitches are recorded clearly. In the film the characteristics of low register are described as follows:

1. thick vocal folds that close firmly for each vibratory cycle
2. a large amplitude of vibration (movement away from the midline)
3. closure and opening of the vocal folds beginning at their lower edges
4. a loud tone rich in harmonic partials (except for the very lowest notes).

The characteristics of high register are shown to be:

1. vocal folds that are stretched thin by the combined action of the crico-thyroids and posterior crico-arytenoids, and at the highest pitches only the vocal ligaments are vibrating (falsetto)
2. glottal closure is brief and incomplete for each cycle because of the high tension in the vocal folds (Fig. 39)
3. the tone has fewer partials and is not as loud as that produced in heavy registration.

In addition to what was shown in the film, in their high register, some singers appear to utilise a little understood phenomenon called damping, in which only a portion of the vocal folds vibrates.

The transition between the two extremes is sometimes considered as separate middle register. Vennard (1970) defines it as a combination of the action of crico-thyroids (as in high falsetto) and the vocalis (as in a medium chest tone) where these two sets of muscles maintain a finely tuned balance. The graduation or transition of register is partially controlled by the contraction of the vocalis on one hand, and on the other, the antagonism of the posterior crico-arytenoids, the lateral crico-arytenoids and the crico-thyroids.

Hirano (1977) has shed further light on registers by studying the physiological and histological properties of the vocal folds which consist of three separate tissues (Fig. 41B) each differing in mechanical properties. These include: the covering of loose and pliant mucosa and the underlying vocal ligament; the transitional or intermediate layer of elastic fibers and dense connective tissue; and the body consisting of the vocalis muscle. Surgeons like Sataloff (2005) have demonstrated further layers of the folds.

Hirano found differences in these three tissues during heavy and light registration. He observed that normally when the crico-thyroids contract, the entire vocal fold becomes stiff due to the longitudinal stretch of all the layers. However when the vocalis muscles contract there is increased thickness of the vocal folds which is directly related to increased loudness in tone. When there is only little or moderate contraction of the vocalis with small pressures, the cover and transitional layers are slackened. When the dominance of the activity of the vocalis over the crico-thyroids prevailed a kind of mucosal wave was seen during heavy registration. On the other hand, when the crico-thyroids exerted greater muscular influence than the vocalis, the vocal folds were stiffened considerably and higher pitches and light registration occurred.

Teachers work hard to help singers make these transitions in registration easily so all the pitches sound with equal quality. When the adjustment of the vocal folds occurs abruptly, a singer will sound as if he has several different voices. The activity of the vocalis muscle is of primary importance because when it does not 'let go' by releasing as the crico-thyroids contract, there is too much muscular antagonism and adjustments become abrupt and jerky leading to breaks in the voice.

When a singer is accused of carrying the chest voice up too high, it means that the vocalis has too much tension in it. This happens because

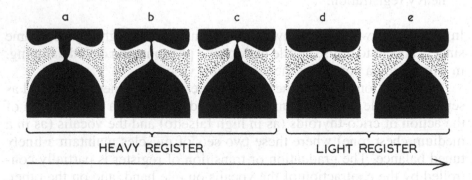

Fig. 44. Registration.
This schematic drawing of the vocal folds (shown in white) shows their shape and position during heavy and light registration. Note: *1* the thickness of the vocal folds for heavy register, also that they touch along a wide area; *2* during light registration they hardly touch and when they do, it is only at the free upper border which is supported by the vocal ligaments. This knowledge is often the key to audible discernment ofthe location of vocal fold pathology such as nodules. If hoarseness is heard only on low register pitches, it is likely that the nodule(s) is located on the lower portion of the vocal fold. Therefore hoarseness heard only in low registers is likely to be due to adverse changes (*e.g.* a nodule) on the lower surface(s) of the fold, if heard only in higher registers this suggests pathological changes in the edge(s) of the fold.

the muscles that help stretch the vocal folds for high pitches and the antagonism of too much strain in the vocal folds and surrounding muscles create a 'tug of war' which leads to the voice cracking or breaking as it moves higher. Singing in a heavy voice in too high a range creates vocal strain, muscle fatigue and, ultimately may lead to the formation of nodules on the vocal folds.

Little is known about the extrinsic laryngeal factors influencing registration. Historically, teachers have helped singers to master the transitions by having them darken or 'cover' the tone as they move to higher registers or to modify the vowel sound. More recently the emphasis on balanced alignment and physical freedom seems to work also. These techniques help create more space and a release in the pharynx and allow the larynx to remain low. Practically this means that the larynx is physically poised in a position where it can vibrate optimally. Whereas on excessively bright or wide open sounds, there is tension in the supra laryngeal muscles causing the larynx to rise, therefore inhibiting efficient vibration.

Generally the main transition point in the female voice is between the heavy and middle, and in the male voice it is between the middle and light registers. Unskilled singers tend to stay in one register without trying to bridge the gap, partly because they mistakenly *perceive* a change in quality as they go from one to another and partly because they are unable to equalise vocal quality. Young singers are influenced by the preponderance of heavy singing in the field of popular music and often find it difficult to appreciate and use the higher pitches in their voices. Initially they may reject the light registration because it does not seem to sound mature and full. So typically, they sing in low keys and avoid the higher registers. With training they can be shown a healthy technique for using the whole compass of their voices and so enrich their performances.

Subglottic pressure and vocal intensity

The good singer begins a sound with prior thought and a proper attack, and at the same time is able to maintain a tone of constant loudness and pitch. Part of this evenness of tone is created by a constant pressure of air just below the vocal folds, the subglottic pressure (see page 84). Two factors are necessary in maintenance of subglottic pressure: (1) the contraction of the adductor muscles of the larynx; and (2) expiratory force (Kirchner, 1970).

When the adductor muscles contract, the opening between the folds is narrowed or even closed; this action increases resistance to the upcoming air and therefore reduces the rate of flow. When the glottal resistance remains constant, then any increased expiratory force will cause the air flow rate to increase. Isshiki (1964) found that at very low pitches the glottal resistance is dominant in controlling intensity (laryngeal control), that it becomes less so as the pitch is raised, and that finally at extremely high pitches the intensity is controlled almost entirely by the rate of flow of air which is then controlled by expiratory muscles. However, when at any pitch level the loudness of the tone is increased, glottal resistance becomes the major factor in supporting that loudness (Rubin et al., 1967).

The control of vocal intensity, pitch, subglottic air pressure and rates of air flow involves a highly complex co-ordination of mechanisms operating within the larynx, the respiratory system and other areas of the body. A study by Rubin, LeCover and Vennard (1967) found that either narrowing of the vocal tract or breathiness had a seriously disturbing effect on the relationship of air flow and subglottic pressure, and poor control of breathing impaired vocal quality. When coordination of all these forces is precise and spontaneous, vocal problems such as breathiness, unevenness of tonal quality, pitch difficulties, wobbles and many more undesirable inefficiencies are eliminated.

Summary

A singer who is well trained has a balanced and spontaneous co-ordination of the vocal attack, air flow and subglottic pressure. Such co-ordination allows the singer to perform with optimum efficiency. This delicate physical balance can be upset by excessive tension or inadequate muscular activity. Too much muscular constriction causes the larynx to be excessively high or exaggeratedly depressed, making the vocal tone sound strained or swallowed; whereas inadequate muscular tension is characterised by a breathy tone, lack of proper intensity and shallowness in the sound. These conditions interfere with efficient singing production by restricting the free vibration of the vocal folds, mainly because the larynx has been physically inhibited by undue muscular constriction or pulled away from its natural position in the neck by misalignment of the head, neck and shoulders.

Titze (1979, 2000) has emphasized the importance of balance of muscular activity within the larynx as well as the role of opposing muscles in efficient vocal production. He suggests that this balance *"maximises vocal efficiency by minimising configurational changes in the dynamics of vocal production. Excessive glottal stops, voice 'breaks', large vertical excursions of the larynx with pitch, and gross movement of the shoulders and rib cage during breathing may be the result of allowing unopposed muscles to strain various tissues to the point of saturation. Such postural and configurational changes, which are often corrected by similar drastic oppositional manoeuvres, could cause undesirable transient acoustic responses, waste energy, and probably contribute to the apparent lack of control in voice production."*

A well trained singer has to go through a seemingly formidable and intimidating checklist. In order to pretune, he must conceive the pitch, quality of tone, and emotion desired, then take an adequate breath with no interfering tension, and attack the tone with clarity and precision. Throughout a song the evenness of vocal quality must be regulated by adjusting the register in the appropriate places in the range, and by balancing the intensity and dynamics of sound in a proper emotional context. Fortunately all this happens at subconscious levels or no singer would be able to function. The ultimate point of study and training is to ensure that these complex co-ordinations become habits so spontaneous that the singer is freed to think about the art of communication with an audience rather than the act of phonation.

8 Resonation and vocal quality

Artistic singing and speaking depend on a person's ability to establish optimum conditions for vocal resonance. When the vocal instrument is capable of free and dynamic response to the demands of the singer, optimum resonance is derived from the singer's image of sound together with what he senses when he makes that sound, the physical response of the muscles of the pharynx and balance with the rest of the body. Vocal pedagogy and the relevant literature relating to vocal quality is fraught with a confusion of communication, scientific terminology and imagery. The difficulties of finding qualitative verbal estimates of sound become apparent the more one reads. Descriptions of tone may include metaphors such as white, spread, harsh, unpleasant, warm, round, full, bright and clear. There is no other way of describing sound unless one uses strictly scientific and mathematical terms, and even then certain vocal qualities defy quantification.

Finding adequate verbal description for teaching a sensory experience can be difficult and teachers and authors often resort to inappropriate imagery. This has led to the problem of confusing sensation with theory and has given rise to many scientifically unfounded descriptions. The idea that singing feels as if it is in the head or in the front of the face (sometimes termed in the mask) does not mean that it is actually happening there. Some writers have complicated matters further by postulating the existence of tones placed in the various sinuses, and drawn diagrams with arrows pointing to anatomical places in the head where one should feel the tone. Such explanations attempt to deal with the sensory aspects of sound by finding a physical place to fit the explanation. However further thought reveals that these contrivances usually cannot be taken literally. Good singers eventually find their own whole body awareness and pattern of sensations that become consistent as they study and practice.

The resonator for increasing sonority in the voice is the vocal tract (Fig. 46); this consists of the larynx, pharynx, and mouth, and on rare

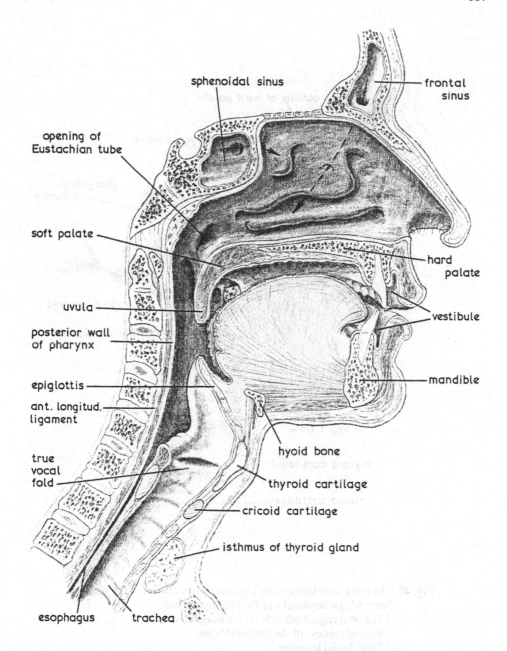

Fig. 45. Sagittal section of the vocal tract.
Note: *1* The nasal pharynx extends from the base of the skull to the soft palate. *2* The oral pharynx includes the space between the soft palate and glosso-epiglottic folds. *3* The laryngeal pharynx extends from the glosso-epiglottic folds to the lower border of the cricoid cartilage.
The positions of the soft palate, tongue, hyoid bone, and larynx vary with muscular action, and therefore, the length and shape of the vocal tract is also variable.

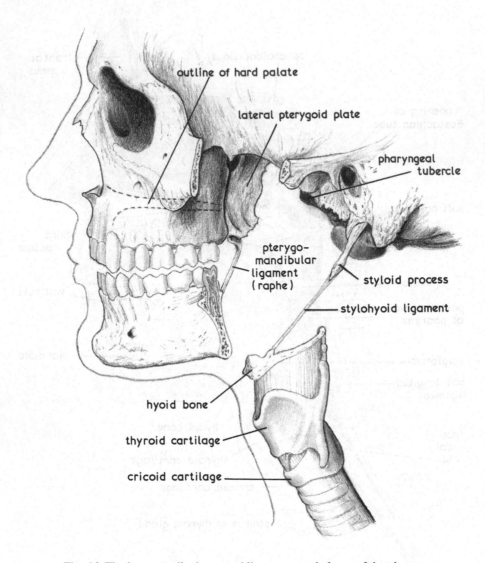

outline of hard palate

lateral pterygoid plate

pharyngeal tubercle

pterygo-
mandibular
ligament
(raphe)

styloid process

stylohyoid ligament

hyoid bone

thyroid cartilage

cricoid cartilage

Fig. 46. The bony, cartilaginous and ligamentous skeleton of the pharynx.
Note: Major landmarks of the pharynx include:
1 The pharyngeal tubercle on the occipital bone
2 Styloid process of the temporal bone
3 Stylo-hyoid ligament
4 Hard palate
5 Lateral Pterygoid plate
6 Pterygomandibular raphé
7 Hyoid bone, body, lesser and greater horns
8 Thyroid cartilage, oblique line, superior and inferior horns
9 Cricoid cartilage

occasions for nasalized sounds, the nose. Because parts of the tract are muscular and highly mobile, it is capable of changes in length and width which alter the resonance of the voice as well as the quality of tone. Paget (1930) observed that the texture of the walls of a resonator also affects quality of tone. Thus, when the walls are relaxed, high frequencies are absorbed and the tone tends to be damped; when the walls are thin and flexible, the sound waves cause them to pulsate and awaken sympathetic vibrations of the air space within the vocal tract.

This chapter explains some details of the vocal tract, very general aspects of the acoustics, and conditions which alter the shape of the resonator and therefore affect formation of vowels and vocal quality. This is a complicated area of voice with much research yet to be done. It is hoped by understanding what information we do have available, the reader will be provided with a firmer basis for analysis of sound so that there is less recourse to speculation. In addition, an informed teacher or student will be wise enough to know that while an individual's bone structure and other physical features of his instrument determines his maximum potential for quality of resonance, that limit is rarely reached in practice. Too many singers are unaware that careful work and training can improve their tonal quality and that many great singers were at one point in their training dismissed as having puny voices.

It is difficult to observe what happens inside a singer while he is performing and therefore many of the changes in the pharynx remain shrouded in mystery. A few X-ray studies by Russell (1931), Sonninen (1964), Damsté (1968), Bunch (1974) and Bunch and Sonninen (1977), and MacCurtain (1981) have shed some light on the topic and there is optimism for the future of Magnetic Resonance Imaging (Stark, 1984; Baker,1986; Hoffman, 1990). As the pharynx is the most important resonator of the voice, it is worthwhile to spend time looking at its anatomical details. Structures that are specifically articulatory in nature are described in Chapter 9.

The anatomy and physiology of the pharynx

The pharynx extends from the base of the skull to the posterior surface of the base of the cricoid cartilage. It has three parts; the nasal pharynx, oral pharynx and laryngeal pharynx. It is a mobile muscular sleeve lined with mucous membrane with four openings (Fig. 46), the paired posterior apertures of the nose and the single oral and laryngeal openings. The oral and upper laryngeal sections of the pharynx serve as an air and food passageway and these two paths cross. The inhaled air must go through the larynx to the lungs, and the food must bypass the larynx to enter the esophagus which begins at the lower border of the cricoid cartilage. During the complex act of swallowing the air passageway is protected. As food moves through the passageway the muscles of the pharynx contract in succession, beginning superiorly. Food is squeezed into the esophagus and thence to the stomach. During swallowing the breath is held, the larynx is pulled upwards and forwards and the vocal folds close tightly to prevent food from entering the trachea and eventually reaching the lungs. On the other hand, for breathing, the pharyngeal muscles must relax to allow adequate passage of air. At that time the glottis is open and the top of the esophagus closed (to prevent air from entering the stomach). Obviously it is unwise to eat and talk at the same time because the resultant protective reflexes are suppressed and may cause air or food to enter the wrong passageway, even then there is the final protective reflex of coughing when liquids or solids stimulate the larynx and trachea.

The pharynx makes an unusual resonator component of the system because it is used for something far removed from singing most of the time and is capable of being altered in shape and form. Depending on the shape of the pharynx and the position of the head, the sound waves from the larynx will be reflected from its walls in a variety of ways.

The three sections of the pharynx are each capable of contributing some kind of resonance. The uppermost section, the nasal pharynx, extends from the base of the skull to the soft palate (Fig. 46) and has a number of noteworthy features:

(1) it can be closed off by the mobile soft palate as in swallowing when food is prevented from entering the nose, and also for the production of certain sounds of speech;

(2) the reason a performer hears his own sound differently from a listener is attributed to the opening into the nasal pharynx of the Eustachian or tympanic tube, and to the conduction of vibrations by bone to the middle and inner ears;

(3) the sinuses and tear ducts open into the nasal cavity and can cause secondary congestion of the nasal mucosa.

The nasal pharynx amplifies nasal consonants and vowels in various languages and in some regional patterns of speech like those in the mountains and mid western areas of the United States and areas of Australia.

The middle or oral section of the pharynx extends from the soft palate to the inlet of the larynx and is the largest of the resonating spaces. Since the palate and larynx are both capable of moving upwards, downwards, forwards and backwards, it is this portion of the pharynx whose shape is the most changeable. Movements and alterations in the shape of the tongue are significant in this section because these can alter the shape of the resonating space and obstruct the aperture of the oral pharynx. The tongue has complex connections to the larynx, pharynx and soft palate (Figs. 46 and 61) and when it contracts, its changes in shape affect the shape of the vocal tract. Also the jaw has connections to this part of the pharynx and its movements can alter sound markedly.

The inferior or laryngeal portion of the pharynx extends from the inlet of the larynx to the base of the cricoid cartilage (Fig. 45). The opening of the larynx, some times called the collar of the larynx, is formed by the epiglottis and ary-epiglottic folds (Fig. 38), and is thought to contribute the area of resonance which gives the voice a ringing quality, often referred to as the *"ring"* in the literature.

The bones and ligaments to which the pharynx is attached are shown in Fig. 46 and the muscles in Fig. 47.

Three important groups of paired muscles contribute to the formation of the pharynx:

a) the constrictors

There are the largest muscles, are arranged circumferentially, and when contracted lessen the width of the pharynx. The superior, middle and inferior constrictors are separate muscles extending from the pharyngeal tubercle to the esophagus and they are placed one inside the other – like stacked flower pots – with the superior constrictor innermost (Fig. 47). During swallowing these muscles function in a smooth sequence beginning with the superior constrictor initiating peristalsis, the reflex muscular wave that sends food through the digestive tract. After passing gus. The constrictors are striated, fast-acting muscle which narrow the through the laryngeal pharynx, swallowed material enters the esophapharyngeal pathway when contracted, an action unfavourable to singing and speaking.

b) the relatively slender longitudinal muscles which shorten the length of the pharynx

There are four paired, slender longitudinal muscles of the pharynx which help to suspend and to elevate the larynx from behind, and therefore they also reduce the length of the pharynx. These are the stylo-hyoids, the stylo-pharyngeus, the palato-pharyngeus and the tiny salpingo-pharyngeus which joins and becomes part of the palato-pharyngeus (Figs. 48 and 49).

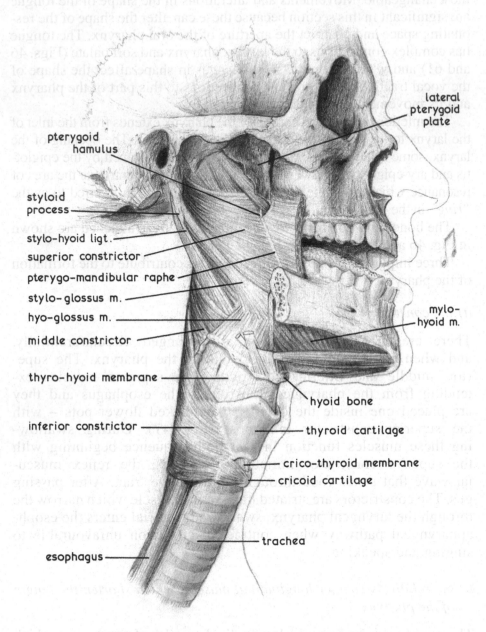

Fig. 47. The constrictors of the pharynx – lateral view.

These are paired muscles, and the figure shows those of the right side.

Each *superior constrictor* arises from the lower portion of the medial pterygoid plate, the pterygomandibular raphé, and from a small area behind the molars on the inside of the mandible. Fibers sweep round posteriorly to be inserted in the pharyngeal raphé on the pharyngeal tubercle in the midline and below that into another raphé or cord also in the midline.

c) The muscles of the soft palate

In order to complete any discussion of the pharynx, the soft palate must be included (even though it is involved in articulation as well). The soft palate may be elevated, tensed or relaxed. Elevation is accomplished by contraction of the levator palati muscles. The tensor palati muscle tenses the palate by pulling it horizontally. Both actions are most important for speech and singing because this creates more resonating space in the oral pharynx and blocks off the nasal pharynx, preventing an undesirable nasal tone. The relaxed soft palate hangs downwards leaving the nasal port open. This leads to an ugly hypo functional vocal production with too much nasal resonance. Figures 48 and 49 show these muscles in detail.

The anatomical and physiological mechanisms of the pharynx are interdependent and extremely complex. The interrelated patterns of movement of the pharynx, soft palate, tongue, larynx and jaw are still being studied and it is clear that this complicated interaction makes it almost impossible to isolate the function of a single muscle (Fig. 50). It is not difficult to understand why the resonating functions of the pharynx are so controversial. Because of the sensitivity of the pharynx, there are few direct studies on live subjects. X-ray has afforded one of the few ways of assessing its function and although expensive, magnetic resonance imaging and ultrasound may pave the way into the future. Most functional studies have approached the problem from an acoustic standpoint (Sundberg, 1977,1985; Cleveland, 1977). This type of research is proving attractive because it is particularly suited to computer analysis. Therefore it is necessary to include a brief account of the acoustics involved in the vocal tract.

Each *middle constrictor* arises from the lower portion of the stylo-hyoid ligament, the lesser horn, and whole length of the greater horn of the hyoid bone. It fans out into a triangle so that the right and left muscles form a diamond shape, and both are attached posteriorly to the pharyngeal raphé.

Each *inferior constrictor* consists of two parts: *1* an upper portion which arises above from the oblique line of the thyroid cartilage, and below from a fibrous arch linking the thyroid and cricoid cartilages together. These fibers are inserted into the pharyngeal raphé; *2* a lower ring-like portion called the *crico-pharyngeus* muscle which arsises from the cricoid cartilage and continues without a raphé to the other side. It forms the superior sphincter of the esophagus which relaxes when solids or liquids reach the lower end of the pharynx.

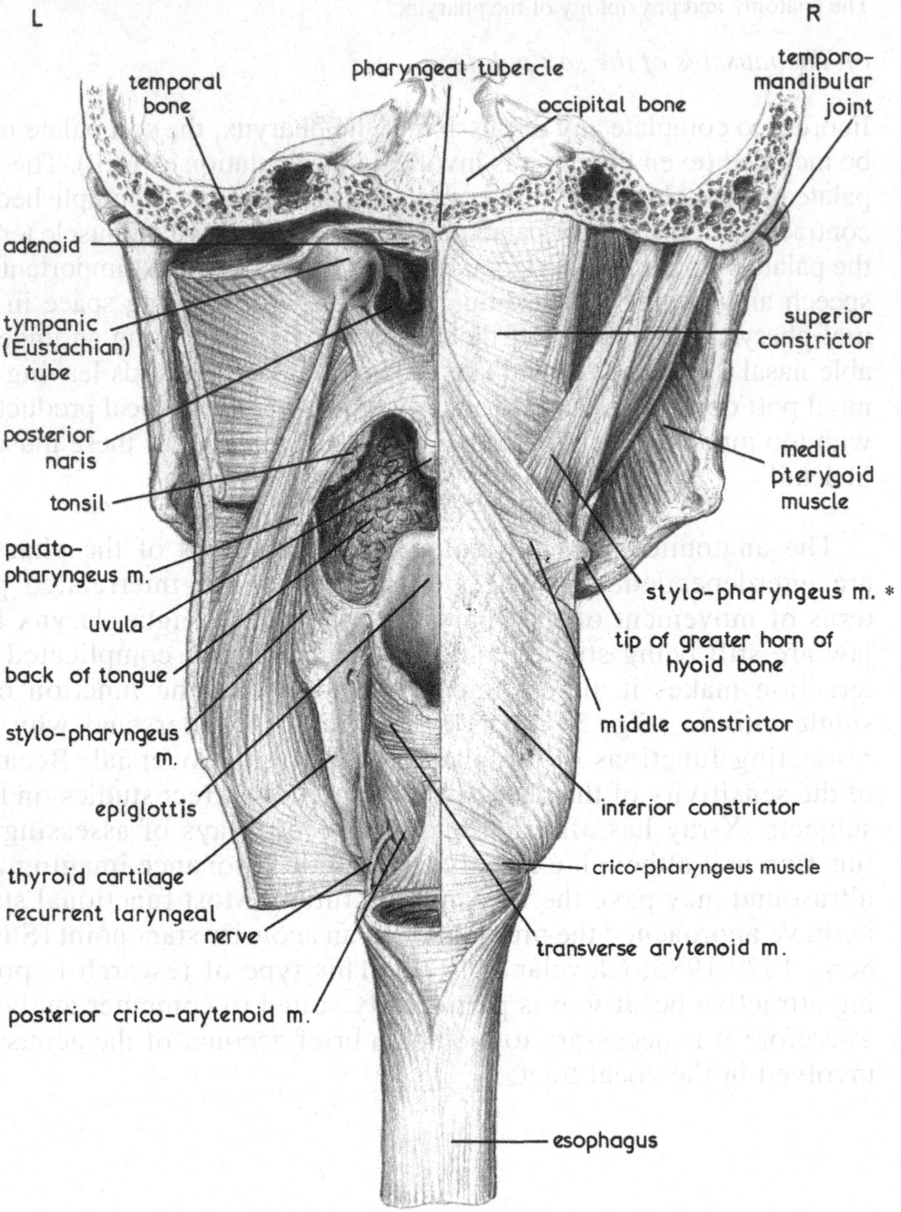

Fig. 48. The longitudinal muscles of the pharynx.
These muscles are also paired and are seen from behind in this figure.
Each *stylo-hyoid* muscle is attached to the styloid process and the lesser horn of the hyoid bone.
The fibers of the *stylo-pharyngeus* run from the styloid process to the superior horn of the thyroid cartilage and the adjacent pharyngeal fascia.
The *palato-pharyngeus* is attached to the soft palate and also the superior horn of the thyroid cartilage and pharyngeal fascia.
The *salpingo-pharyngeus* is a tiny slip of muscle that is attached to the cartilaginous end of the tympanic tube (Eustachian) and joins the fibers of palato-pharyngeus.

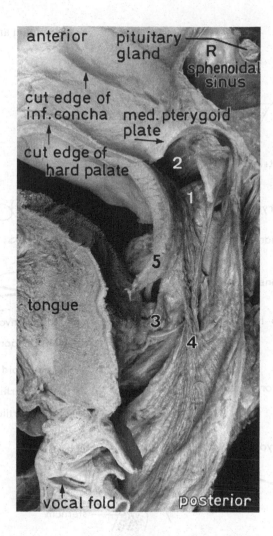

Fig. 49. The muscles of the soft palate on the right side and viewed from the medial surface in the mouth.

(By kind permission of the Anatomy Department of the Royal College of Surgeons of England.)

Each *levator veli palatini (1)* is attached to the base of the skull (petrous portion of the temporal bone) and the inferior surface of the cartilagenous portion of the tympanic tube, and the tendons spread out and merge with that of the other side in the soft palate, which they elevate.

Tensor veli palatini (2) arises from the scaphoid fossa (between the pterygoid plates) and tympanic tube, the delicate cylindrical tendon hooks round a process of the medial pterygoid plate, pierces buccinator and then spreads out and is attached to the posterior border of the hard palate as well as merging with the palatine aponeurosis. It tenses the soft palate, and opens the tympanic tube thus equalizing the air pressure in the tube, middle ear and pharynx during swallowing.

Palato-glossus (3) arises from the soft palate and passes downwards to be inserted posteriorly into the side of the tongue.

Palato-pharyngeus (4) arises from the soft palate and is inserted on the superior horn of the thyroid cartilage and pharyngeal fascia.

The *uvula (5)* covers a pair of tiny muscles extending from either side of the midline of the posterior border of the hard palate, and it contributes to closure of the nasal pharynx.

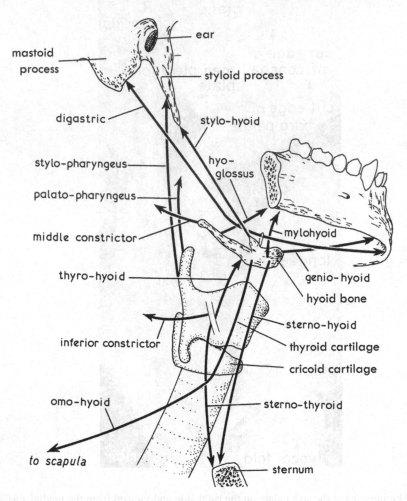

Fig. 50. Diagram of lines of pull of the constrictors of the pharynx and other muscles steady-
ing and supporting the larynx (right side only shown).
The complexities and interrelationships of the muscles of the head and neck make it difficult
to readily assess definitive muscle action in speech and singing. However, it can be clearly
shown here that changes in position of the larynx, pharynx and tongue inevitably affect the
shape of the vocal tract.

A summary of the acoustics of the vocal tract[1]

When a person wishes to sing, expiratory air flow through the vocal folds
and the subsequent opening and closing of the vocal folds create pulsation in the glottal air stream which give the fundamental frequency.[2]
The fundamental frequency in speech and singing is changing all the
time, however components of laryngeal tone are always harmonics of

the fundamental and the *"effects of the resonances of the vocal tract is to produce a peak in the spectrum (Fig. 51) of the output of the harmonics which are closest to the true resonance. This ensures that the spectrum always has the same general outline as well as the sameness in quality in a range of sounds with different fundamentals"* (Fry, 1979).

The relationship of the wave length of the sounds created by the vocal folds to the dimensions of the vocal tract (air column) is the key to the phenomenon of resonance. This is complicated because no two wave lengths are the same size and shape, and short-term changes in the vocal tract are brought about by articulatory movements (Fry, 1979). In addition to the unevenness of shape and movements of the vocal tract, the materials of which it is made are muscles and surface tissues which are all relatively soft and consequently damp the sound and absorb more energy. This is explained by Winckel (1967):

"Resonant vibration can arise in a hollow body if its walls are excited or if a vibrating air column of the resonant frequency of the hollow body is permitted to enter through an opening. When the inner surface is hard as metal, the resonance is sharp; if it is covered with an absorbent coating, the resonance is less sharp and the resonance curve is broader. The damping of the soft inner surface of the human mouth causes larger losses through absorption than the hard inner surface of a violin body" (Fig. 52).

He further states:

"Such hollow bodies are called Helmholtz resonators. The frequency range in which overtones from the sound source receive a reaction depends on the size and to some extend on the shape of hollow body. The sound of the human voice yields a spectrum whose components result from a number of cavities: pharynx, oral cavity, nasal cavity and windpipe."

Thus the supra laryngeal airway serves as an acoustic filter which, depending on the shape and stiffness of its walls, can suppress some of the sound energy at certain frequencies while allowing maximum sound energy or formant frequencies to pass through. The shape and stiffness of the vocal tract will vary individually according to the amount of relaxation or tension present, and in the case of laryngeal cartilages, age may bring about calcification and even ossification. Therefore there will be slight individual differences in acoustic (spectral) patterns from singer to

---

[1] Detailed acoustics of the vocal tract may be found in such texts as those by Winckel (1967), Fry (1979), Sundberg (1987) and Titze (1994).
[2] Fundamental frequency is defined as the rate of opening and closing of the vocal folds, or pitch.

singer. However, the recognition of tonal character and establishment of tonal colour are due to pronounced resonance peaks in the spectrum of partials. These peaks are given the name of formants. Strictly speaking, a formant is a range of frequencies, but since a formant must give rise to a peak in the spectrum of sound produced, the term formant is commonly applied to the frequency at which this peak occurs (Fry, 1979). Formants are the most significant earmarks of sound, and every vowel is formed by two or more formant ranges. A discussion of vowels follows on pages 130–139.

The formation or the strength of formant frequencies depends on the relationship of the vibrating frequency of the vocal folds to the resonating frequency of the pharynx and further depends on the amount of damping[3]. For example, it is possible for only odd numbered overtones to respond thus yielding a hollow-sounding tone colour. For this reason it is easier to imitate synthetically the sounds of brass instruments than those of the voice. When there is severe damping of resonances in the vocal tract there are wider resonance curves for the formants, and therefore a wider excitation zone for the formation of the non-harmonic partials (Winckel, 1967). In other words when the walls of the pharynx absorb too much sound, there is more scope for a tonal quality that is not desired.

According to Sundberg (1977) there are four or five important formants. The first four peaks occur in the regions of 500, 1500, 2500 and 3500 cycles (or Hertz) per second respectively. These formants will shift areas (i.e. 500 to 550) according to the various conformations of the vocal tract (Fig. 53). The fifth formant important to singing, labelled the "ring" of the voice by Vennard (1967), occurs between 2500 and 3200 Hertz. It is thought to result from the lengthening of the vocal tract (Fig. 54A). Sundberg (1977) explains this formant in the following way:

"The insertion of an extra formant between the normal third and fourth formants would produce the kind of peak that is seen in the spectrum of a sung vowel. Moreover, the acoustics of the vocal tract when the larynx is lowered are compatible with the generation of such an extra formant. It can be calculated that if the area of the outlet of the larynx into the pharynx is less than a sixth of the area of the cross section of the pharynx, then the larynx is acoustically mismatched with the rest of the vocal tract: it has a resonance frequency of its own, largely dependent of the remainder of the tract."

Sundberg and others acknowledge that the lowering of the larynx also explains major differences of vowel quality in speech and singing.

---

[3] Not to be confused with the damping that occurs in the larynx on high pitches.

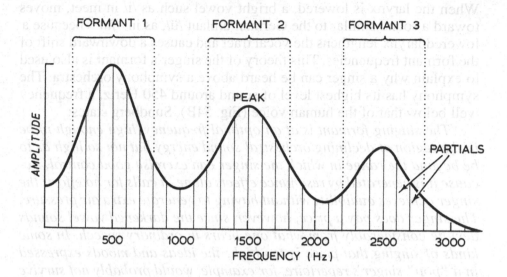

Fig. 51. Schematic drawing of a sound spectrum of the vocal tract.
The sound spectrum represents the spectrum of resonance frequencies of which human vocal sound is composed. The frequencies are set out on the horizontal scale in Hertz (cycles per second). Each vertical line is equal to a partial or overtone which is a harmonic of the fundamental (pitch). Note: some partials are much stronger than others. The reinforcement or strength of some overtones gives the differences in quality of sound such as the specific characteristics of vowel sound and/or type of instrument being played. The resonance frequencies give rise to peaks in the spectrum which are termed formants. The formant structure is the basis for the recognition of different vowels.

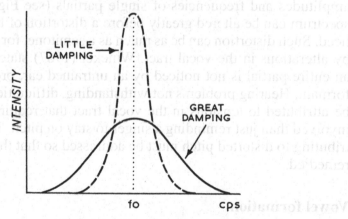

Fig. 52. Schematic spectrum of damped sound.
Damped sound is the result of absorption or reflection of sound energy. As shown here damped sound (which has the same pitch as the undamped) has a frequency curve that is less sharp or steep than a sound with little or no damping. In the singer, damping is caused by the changing shape and thickness of the walls of the resonator(s).

When the larynx is lowered, a bright vowel such as /i/ in meet, moves toward a sound similar to the German umlaut /ü/, as in *"für"* because a lowered larynx lengthens the vocal tract and causes a downward shift of the formant frequencies. This theory of the singer's formant is also used to explain why a singer can be heard above a symphony orchestra. The symphony has its highest level of sound around 450 Hertz, a frequency well below that of the human voice (Fig. 54B). Sundberg states:

"The singing formant is at an optimal frequency, high enough to be in the region of declining orchestral sound energy but not so high as to be beyond the range in which the singer can exercise good control. Because it is generated by resonance effects alone, it calls for no effort: the singer achieves audibility without having to generate extra air pressure. The singer does pay a price, however, since the darkened vowel sounds deviate considerably from what one hears in ordinary speech. In some kinds of singing that price is too high: the ideas and moods expressed in a "pop" singer's repertoire, for example, would probably not survive the deviations from naturalness that are required to generate the singing formant. And pop singers do not in fact darken their vowels; they depend on electronic amplification to be heard".

Changes in the shape of the vocal tract will alter resonances and inevitably pitch. Such alterations may account for out-of-tune singing by a singer who may have conceived the correct pitch. Some singers become overly conscious of making the correct pitch, and by trying to physically adjust the vocal tract cause excess muscular tension, and therefore create their own pitch problems (see p. 106). However, it is of interest that amplitudes and frequencies of single partials (see Fig. 51) of a sound spectrum can be altered greatly before a distortion of tone colour is noticed. Such distortion can be as much as a semitone, for example, created by alterations in the vocal tract. Winckel (1967) stated that erasure of an entire partial is not noticed by an untrained ear, provided it is not a formant. Hearing problems not withstanding, difficulties with pitch may be attributed to tensions in the vocal tract that require solutions more involved than just reminding a singer to stay on pitch. The tensions contributing to distorted pitch must be addressed so that the problem can be remedied.

Vowel formation

In all languages the phonetic quality of vowels is due to resonances in the vocal tract created mainly by changes in the position of the tongue and to a lesser extent by the lips. As the tongue shifts into different positions, thereby changing the shape of the resonating chamber, resonances

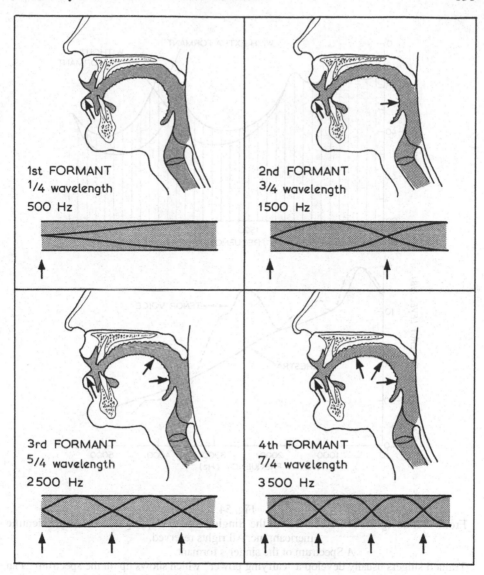

1st FORMANT
1/4 wavelength
500 Hz

2nd FORMANT
3/4 wavelength
1500 Hz

3rd FORMANT
5/4 wavelength
2500 Hz

4th FORMANT
7/4 wavelength
3500 Hz

Fig. 53. The shape of the vocal tract and resulting formants.
(This redrawn diagram is used by kind permission of Sundberg and the editors of Scientific American, 1977.) Alterations in the configuration of the vocal tract gives rise to variations in ranges of formant frequencies. Changes in the frequencies are brought about by different patterns of articulation; these include combinations of variations in the shape and extent of opening of lips, the position of the tongue, mandible and soft palate. The length and cross section of the vocal tract or resonating tube are subjected to changes and these account for varying formants. Each sound, whatever the pitch, has at least four identifiable formants. The diagram illustrates four. Below each drawing through the midline of the vocal tract there is a theoretical diagram of the behavior of sound waves in the tract.

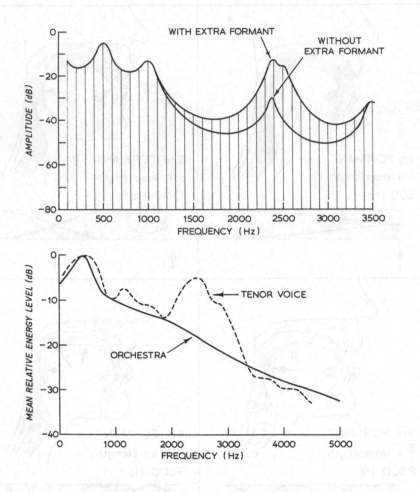

Fig. 54.

A Spectrum of the singer's formant.

Trained singers usually develop a "carrying power" which shows up on the spectrum as an added formant, usually in the frequency range of 2800–3200 Hertz. This formant is often described as the "ring" of the voice.

B Average sound levels of singer and orchestra.

This graph demonstrates the audibility of the trained singer whose optimum frequency is above that of the orchestra.

are either enhanced or damped producing the formant frequencies of vowels (Fig. 55).

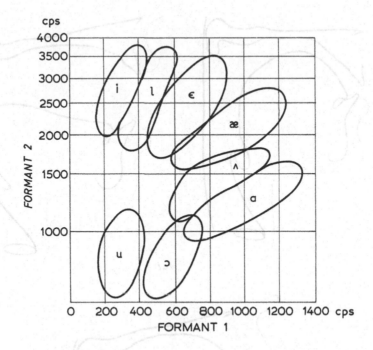

Fig. 55. Ranges of formants for common vowel sounds used in the English language. The first two formants have been utilized in making this diagram of ranges of frequencies of some vowels. The symbols representing the vowel sounds are those of the International Phonetic Alphabet.

There are many books are concerned with the phonetics and descriptions of spoken vowels (and consonants). However, differences occur when vowels are sung, partially because of the extended range of pitch used in singing compared with that of speaking (Fig. 56). A singer ascending a scale requires certain shifts of resonance which are usually achieved by a modification of the vowel sound (see discussion on registers in chapter 7) or it can become shrill or too bright. On the highest pitches, most vowels are modified towards an /a/ (as in father) or /ʌ/ (as in up) to create more resonating space in the pharynx.

A singer who makes a conscious effort to maintain the same vowel colour throughout the range by monitoring that vowel aurally, actually produces for the hearer an uneven quality of vowel as she/he moves through the various registers of the voice. What the listener hears in such a voice as it ascends or descends the scale are changes in quality which, when exaggerated, sound as if a different person begins to sing

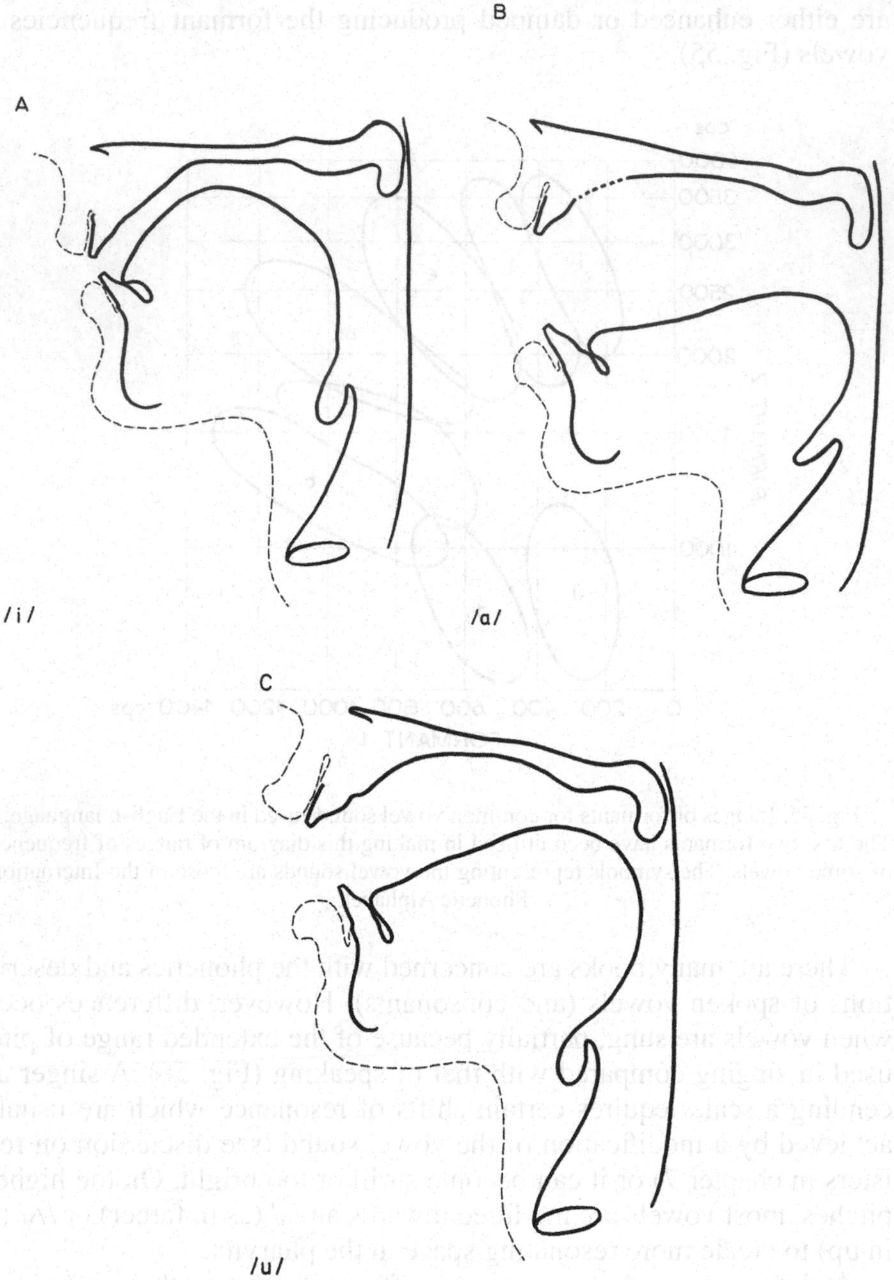

Fig. 56. Tracings made from X-rays of a single individual singing the vowels /i/, /a/ and /u/. These vowels were sung at a pitch of approximately 440 Hertz. Note changes in: the aperture of the mouth, position of the lips, shape of the tongue, and resultant alterations in the shape of the vocal tract. The significance of the minor changes in the shape of the soft palate is unknown.

in each register or in different areas of the range. Winckel (1967) has pointed out that "the tone colour of musical instruments and the human voice changes with the pitch, the tone *colour becoming brighter with ascending pitch*. In addition the vowel colour begins to lose clarity because as the pitch ascends, the functioning area of the lower formant of that vowel is gradually left behind. Winckel (1967) cites as an example the soprano voice that ascends to the level of c3 where the voice will be able to simulate only the formants of the bright vowels. To produce appropriate vowel sounds, constant, small but significant adjustments[4] have to be made in the shape of the resonator. This means that the singer needs to allow pharyngeal space for the sound by having a high soft palate and a comfortably low larynx (Bunch and Sonninen, 1977). Without a dynamic muscular balance between the palate and larynx, the tone can become either pharyngeal or too damped and lose its high frequencies. On the other hand, when this space is not maintained the sound tends to spread or *"whiten"* as the singer ascends the scale, and the number of low frequencies in the sound becomes inadequate for good tonal quality (see page). The effects of various adjustments of the pharynx can be compared to tuning the dials of a stereo system to increase either high or low sound frequencies.

Formation of proper vowel sounds requires little or no movement of the lower jaw and lips (a notable exception is the /u/ and y in German and French), however beginners tend to overlook this and include much too much jaw movement. Ideally, the singer will allow the muscles which elevate the mandible, such as the temporalis (see page), to maintain its balance which will in turn free the tongue to move as needed and the soft palate to remain high.

The basic Italian vowels used in singing are /a/, /e/, /i/, /o/ and /u/ (International Phonetic Alphabet). All additional vowel sounds are modifications of the above; and in order to be proficient in the variety of languages and styles required today; singers must practice all vowels, not only the basic Italian ones.

The lips are able to articulate all vowels efficiently when they are free and relaxed. Lips drawn tightly over the teeth will absorb vibrations and dampen the tone. Lips held in the *"smiling"* position tend to become tense and produce too bright a sound. Because singing will magnify errors made in speech, teachers will find it necessary to spend a considerable amount of time correcting student's vowels.

---

[4] This gradual and controlled modification in the shape of the pharynx and level of the soft palate has been variously described as "covering" or modification of vowel sounds. There has been and is argument about these terms, it is important to understand the basic anatomical changes and their acoustic consequences.

Vocal quality

Vocal quality is the element of singing which initially attracts the listener's attention and determines whether he wishes to hear more. There are four major components of vocal quality: the physical structure of the head, neck and vocal tract, the co-ordination of the mechanism for singing, the imagination of the singer and the levels of health and energy. The most musically proficient student must be born with favourable physical characteristics if she/he hopes to become a great singer. Ideally the bony structures of the head are reasonably symmetrical (but there are often minor variations). A high, wide dental arcade allows maximum space for resonance, and the shape and length of the vocal tract including the palate, and size and length of the vocal folds, all help to determine potential quality. The truly great singer is likely to be well endowed in these respects. The efficient co-ordination and health of the various alterable and unalterable parts of the vocal instrument are requisite for the ultimate good quality of sound.

Even those singers well endowed by nature must then bend efforts to vocal training and giving freedom to their imagination. With patient and conscientious work almost anyone can improve his or her vocal quality and develop the potential for personal optimum sound.

Factors which affect vocal quality

As already indicated, the most favourable conditions of the pharynx for optimum vocal quality are an elevated soft palate, comfortably low larynx, relaxed tongue, and a sense of balance rather than tension in the neck and chest (Fig. 57). Muscular over-reaction to what they are trying to accomplish causes singers the greatest trouble. An experienced teacher can look at a singer in action and predict the quality that will result by noting whether any of several observable signs of tension are present. Six major areas of such tension are discussed below.

(1) Overly active facial muscles

Wrinkled brows, looks of worry or a fixed stare are certainly indicative of a tone that lacks freedom. To demonstrate the effect of tension of the facial muscles around the lips, one can experiment by holding a tone while manipulating the lips and noting the changes in the quality of the tone. A smile or grimace with the lips pulled tightly across the teeth usually brightens the tone until it borders on a white, shallow, straight sound devoid of overtones and vibrato. Some contraltos or basses actually cover the teeth with the lips ostensibly to increase the tonal depth and the tone becomes dark and muffled resulting in a sound that is big

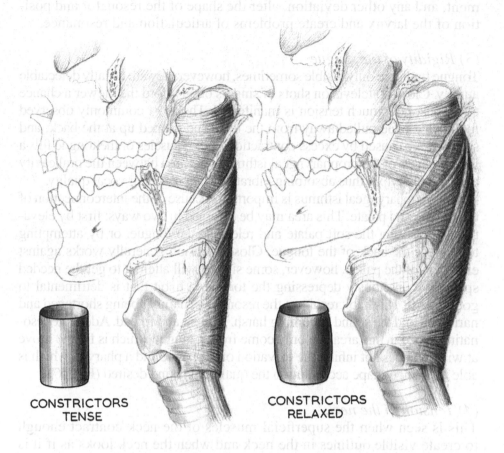

CONSTRICTORS
TENSE

CONSTRICTORS
RELAXED

Fig. 57. Schematic drawing of tensed and relaxed pharynx.

only to the singer, not to the listener. Singers tend to try to use the lips to create changes in the oral cavity; they think that this makes the sound easy to manipulate but in fact they are creating a distortion of the desired quality. Typically the frequencies (either high or low depending on the position of the lips) of the sound become damped and the resulting quality lacks fullness. The singer's face needs never be contorted while singing; rather approach a natural look with the lips relaxed ready to help in articulation.

(2) The position and movement of the lower jaw

Singers (aspiring students and those in the field of pop music particularly) may have the rather common speech habit of protruding the lower jaw rather than lowering it (discussion of the anatomy and function of the lower jaw can be found in Chapter). In singing, this forward displacement, and any other deviation, alter the shape of the resonator and position of the larynx and create problems of articulation and resonance.

(3) Rigidity of the tongue

Tongue faults are only visible sometimes, however they are usually detectable aurally. Close-up television shots of singers often afford the viewer a chance to see just how much tension is manifested. The most commonly observed fault is a tongue pulled away from the teeth and heaped up at the back; and such a lump caused by excess contraction of the muscles of the tongue fills a large volume of the oropharyngeal isthmus (that area between the oral cavity and oral pharynx), thus absorbing vibrations and reducing vocal quality.

The oropharyngeal isthmus is important because of the interconnection of the tongue and palate. This area may be enlarged in two ways: first by elevation and tensing the soft palate and releasing the tongue, or by attempting to depress the back of the tongue. Glossal tension generally works against elevation of the palate, however, some singers will attempt to get the needed space by consciously depressing the tongue, a habit that is detrimental to good sound. This habit results in the resonating chamber being shortened and narrowed and the sound becoming harsh, strident and forced. Adequate resonating space in this area can only come from a tongue which is free to move at will and does not inhibit the elevation of the palate and a pharynx which is able to change shape according to the quality of sound desired (Fig. 57).

(4) Tension in the neck

This is seen when the superficial muscles of the neck contract enough to create visible outlines in the neck and when the neck looks as if it is shrinking in the area just above the larynx. When the contraction is great enough and there is enough pressure below the larynx, the veins will also show. Such over use of muscles tends to displace the larynx and therefore alter the shape of the vocal tract (Fig. 58).

(5) Tension in the chest

When a person has a concave chest and shoulders that are rounded forward, it causes considerable inhibition of the sound, and in particular, loudness. Such tension can be created by out-of-breath singers who try to squeeze more air out of the lungs. Usually it is simply a manifestation of poor postural habits or faulty techniques of breathing.

(6) Emotional tension

Many emotional difficulties will manifest physically and working with the physical aspects of emotion may lead to solving these problems in other areas. Not only does real emotional strain hinder the singer, emo-

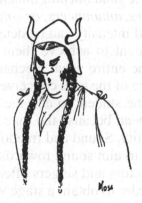
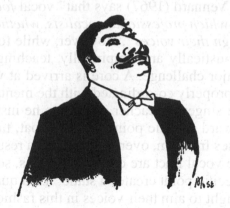

Fig. 58. Caricatures depicting visible tensions which affect vocal quality.
(By kind permission of Librarie Maloine, Paris, from *La Voix,* 1953.)
Note on each singer: the position of the lips, the tension in the face and neck as well as the unnatural position of the head on the neck, and the rigid chest.

tion manufactured to create a more sympathetic performance can also be a drawback. An audience may be moved enough to weep, however when the singer is equally affected, the vocal technique can be seriously impeded. A singer's emotional and physical health is reflected in his/her vocal quality. (See Chapter).

Focus[5] and intensity

A voice unhampered by physical tensions provides a good basis for proper quality of sound. The singer must also concentrate on two additional factors that affect quality: focus, the factor of the sound that maintains a core or centre, and intensity, that element which provides the proper amount of brightness. These are especially important for the singer of concerts and opera and can be observed acoustically by the presence of the singer's formant, the *"ring"*, and certain overtones and wave forms. When the sound is properly intense and focused, it will be heard as a clear precise core around which the tone is centred.

---

[5] Vennard (1967) has described focus as having two aspects, one involving a good attack and clear tone, the other a resonance concept of brilliance. He makes it clear that the term is not to be taken literally but that it indicates to the singer where the most energy is sensed in the vocal tract.

Vennard (1967) says that" vocal *focus is the fundamental dimension by which professional vocalists, whether actors, announcers, or singers, align their voices"*. However, while focus and intensity can be detected acoustically and empirically, teaching a student to achieve them is a major challenge. A core is arrived at when the entire vocal mechanism is properly co-ordinated with the mental image of the tone conceived by the singer. A teacher errs when he instructs the student to aim the tone toward specific points in the throat, face or head because the tone then loses freedom, overtones, and as a result, quality. Sound and freedom in the vocal tract are dynamic entities, so to try to aim sound towards one specific point creates a static, fixed quality. Actors and singers often are taught to aim their voices in this fashion in order to obtain a stage voice quickly. This method is especially reprehensible when applied to the young voice because when the student is finally corrected he is reluctant to relinquish his "*mature*" sounding voice in order to learn a new and proper approach. However, the student must be helped to understand that if he continues to force the tone, he will limit vocal range and quality, eventually inducing vocal strain and fatigue.

Because inexperienced singers are likely to give carrying power (in theatre the term *projection* is often used) to voices by constricting the vocal tract and making a sound that is throaty or resembling a yell, teachers will often direct students to sense the sound some where else such as the head or face in order to avoid such abuse. In some instances such imagery of singing forward and in the head can evoke sensations of freedom in the throat and allow the sound to be released, however the danger of this imagery is that directing the sound forward and in the head can also cause unintentional constriction of the back of the throat. Another difficulty lies in the student's concept of such imagery. No satisfactory definition or scientific investigations have been given for this imagery, yet it is traditional and sometimes practical in teaching.

The best most teachers can do is to refer their students either to areas accessible to vibratory response in the mouth or throat, or to imaginary areas in the closed spaces of the head or consider the option of working more with the physical balance of the body which tends to encourage the natural occurance of focus and clarity of sound. The teacher has to rely on a very fine aural perception in order to guide the student who is by trial and error finding the desired quality. Each singer has a different physiognomy and therefore a slightly different *sense* of focus. This is why teachers need to understand the relationship between physical balance and sound. As the student achieves a certain amount of vocal freedom and co-ordination of the various parts of the vocal mechanism, as well as a good mental concept of the sound, proper focus will result.

Perkins (1977,1978) has made an admirable attempt to address the problem of describing the sensations felt by speakers and singers. Drawing on the fact that professional vocalists describe their techniques in behavioural terms or imagery, Perkins has postulated that the voice is regulated by six independent dimensions; three relate to pitch, loudness and mode, and three relate specifically to the quality of voice: namely constriction, vertical focus and horizontal focus. His views regarding quality are quoted *in extenso* below.

"The feeling of openness of the throat is the perception *by which constriction is regulated along a continuum from open to closed. The closed end is identified reflexively by the peak of a swallow, the open end by the feeling of expansion in the laryngopharynx (throat) at the initiation of a yawn."*

"The other dimension fundamental to vocal efficiency and hygiene is vertical focus. This is the perception associated with the placement of the focal point of the tone in the head. It is the feeling of the location of the focal point of the tone. Although for artistic purposes, especially of the singer at high pitches, a seventh dimension of horizontal focus is important (i.e. where the tone is focused along a continuum from the front to the back of the head) ... At the low end of the focus (vertical) continuum, the tone feels as though it is being squeezed out of the throat. At the high end, the tone seems to float in the head as though it were disconnected from the throat. Focus, like pitch, can be measured on a scale from low to high, but focus and pitch are distinctly separate dimensions of vocal production. Focus of the tone can be moved up or down without changing pitch. Similarly, pitch can be moved up or own without changing focus." [6]

Teachers generally agree that tone produced with a sense of space and ease in the head rather than directing attention to the throat, eliminates constriction of the vocal tract and relieves the larynx of strain and tension allowing it to vibrate freely. The tone produced or focused in the throat involves too much muscular constriction, is of poor quality, and over a period of time will cause enough strain to the vocal folds to create a muscular fatigue and/or pathological changes in the folds. This undesirable method of singing is particularly common to rock, cabaret, and discotheque singers, and their resultant problems provide a busy practice for many laryngologists.

---

[6] Perkins has used the word Perception. He is not referring to physical phenomena.

Some misconceptions regarding resonance

A discussion of resonation would be incomplete without consideration of some popular misconceptions. For example, singers will feel vibrations in the air spaces and bones of the head, and many of these spaces, such as the sinuses, play little or no part in the vocal resonance that is actually perceived by an audience. However, such vibrations do play an important part in the singer's own perception of his/her sound; and this is where the confusion arises. What is actually happening and what the singer is feeling are two different things although they are often treated as one and the same. Research by Russell (1964) and Blanton and Biggs (1968) has shown that the sinuses add little real value to the sound quality, yet the literature is filled with references about the sinuses as major resonators of the voice. Many teachers are thus misled into giving the various sinus cavities of the head undue credit for resonance.

The sinuses do not fulfil the definition of a resonator very well, because they are lined with a mucous membrane that is sound absorbing and their openings are very small (Fig. 59.) Research by Vennard (1964) included having singers' sinuses injected with a harmless solution and then singing in a recital hall. Recordings taken of singing with unfilled and filled sinuses were analysed and showed no significant differences in resonance. Therefore he concluded that the vibrations felt in these areas by the singer are not carried in the form of audible resonance or vocal quality. The teacher who understands this distinction will be able to explain the need for students to separate sensation from function.

Preliminary investigation of the acoustic properties of the nasal tract has been made by Lindquist-Gauffin and Sundberg (1976). Their study involved specific nasalized sounds, seldom utilised in English and Italian, and they postulated that sinus resonance was linked to those sounds, however more extensive studies are yet to be published.

When the nose and sinuses really make no significant contribution to resonance there is the problem of why the speaking voice is so radically altered when one has a cold and/or sinusitis, and the singing voice is unchanged or only slightly altered. One hypotheses might be that in speaking the congestion and swollen mucous membranes help to create a lazy palatal action thereby causing hyper nasality, whereas in singing the performer makes a greater effort to lift the palate (sometimes described as singing *"over a cold"*).

The nose is another of those areas where the singer feels vibrations that are not discerned by the audience unless a nasal consonant or vowel is intended and deliberately produced. For true nasal resonance to occur air must escape through the nose, and if the palate is elevated this is most unlikely.

However the roof of the mouth is the floor of the nose and this might possibly explain the sensation since the mouth is always involved in resonation.

While it would be comforting for singers and teachers to find such a definite place as the nose or a particular sinus where the sound could be placed each time one sang, the fact remains that every singer is physically unique, therefore each singer has to develop (by trial and error and help from his teacher) his/her own set of clear, reproducible sensations in order to stabilize the vocal technique.

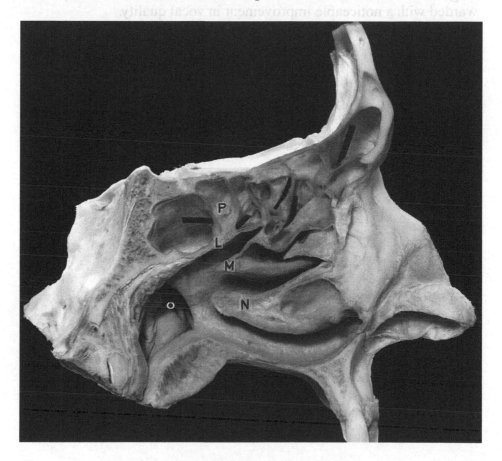

Fig. 59. Left lateral wall of the nasal cavity.
(By kind permission of the Anatomy Department of the Royal College of Surgeons of England.) Note: 1. The bony projections into the cavity (eg. M and N) which are covered with vascular mucous membrane. This produces an increased surface area for warming, moistening and cleaning the inspired air. 2. The black rods are placed in the openings between the paranasal sinuses and nasal cavity. These openings are tiny and covered with mucous membrane. 3. The opening (o) of the tympanic (Eustacian) tube into the nasal pharynx.

Conclusion

Because the vocal tract is so complex anatomically and acoustically, many problems about sensation and vocal quality remain unanswered. There is unquestionable evidence that in singing the vocal tract must be free to respond dynamically by being spacious and without constriction, which will in turn allow the tone to achieve optimal resonance; and the singer who bends his efforts to these ends will almost certainly be rewarded with a noticeable improvement in vocal quality.

Articulation 9

Singing is a unique way of communicating the ideas and emotions of writers and poets. The performer who cannot articulate the words of a song so that they are understood has defeated the whole purpose of his art (unless he is singing one of the rare songs without words). The specific way of articulating sounds varies from language to language. Therefore a careful study of all the languages to be sung is important, especially since no one cares to hear his own language pronounced poorly, even by foreigners. In addition, since movements of articulatory structures like the tongue, lower jaw, soft palate and lips directly influence the shape of the resonator, faulty diction and inefficient articulation inevitably impoverish tonal quality.

Reports of research in the fields of speech, linguistics and phonetic science abound, dealing with almost all of the facets of articulation such as movements of the soft palate, tongue and lips. A large body of work dedicated to the study of congenital cleft palate and/or lip as well as other articulatory defects has contributed to our knowledge about both normal and abnormal movement of the articulatory structures. However, the above studies and reports usually ignore the particular problems of articulation as it relates to singing. The records of research into standard articulatory movements in different languages can be found in any good text of physiology of speech or phonetics.

Vowels and consonants: a summary

a) Vowels

Vowels are shaped and formed in the vocal tract by the tongue and to a lesser extent, the lips. The student of singing is usually surprised to learn that the production of vowels and most consonants requires little active movement of the lower jaw. Provided the muscles elevating the jaw are properly balanced, the tongue will do most of the work without interference or antagonism from the muscles of mastication (see page 150).

There are a variety of diction books in various languages which are specifically directed toward the singer's needs. Phonetics books, mainly concerned with speaking, are helpful for consonants and understandably omit the differences in singing vowels on high pitches because of the associated vowel modification and covering mentioned in Chapter 8.

Many singers who think they are enunciating clearly are guilty of strange and unnecessary labial gymnastics. The lips require no drastic changes for vowel formation. In fact singers often are advised to think of 'imploding' rather than exploding vowels and consonants. Retraction of the lips or smiling is not essential for vowel formation, yet this is a common practice with the neophyte singer. A student with this habit generates a sound that is mouthy and bright, particularly for the vowels /i/ and /e/. When these vowels are produced this way they then do not match the other vowels in colour and quality.

Diphthongs are a gliding complex of vowel sounds and may be double or triple. 'Collins Dictionary of the English Language' defines the terms this way: *"A vowel sound, occupying a single syllable, during the articulation of which the tongue moves from one position to another, causing a continual change in vowel quality, as in pronunciation of a in English late, during which the tongue moves from the position of /e/ towards /ɪ/."* They are physically produced as separate vowel sounds, which are not given equal duration. For example, the word 'night' has the diphthong /ai/, the sounds /a/ (father) and /ɪ/ (sit). The difference in production is that the /a/ sound is more important and therefore sustained for a longer period of time.

b) Consonants

The production of consonants must be crisp, quick and efficient (imploded rather than exploded) so that a singer's performance and quality of tone has proper clarity and meaning. Consonants are classified according to their physical construction and to the presence or absence of laryngeal sound. They may be voiced or voiceless, for example, s is voiceless, z is voiced. Figure 60 is a table summarised from Wise (1958) but differing somewhat in exact classifications.

A careful look at this chart will show that it is the tongue and lips that do most of the work of articulation. Only for sounds such as sh, j, ch, s, and z need one consider closing the mouth. The singer who tries to articulate by excessive motion of the lower jaw in effect changes his or her resonator for each sound. The result is poor diction, unsatisfactory resonance and a muddled garbled sound.

Class of Sound	Anatomical Area	Examples	
		Voiced	Voiceless
Bilabial	Upper and lower lips	b, m*	p
Labiodental	Upper teeth and lower lip	v	f
Dental	Upper teeth and tongue	q (thing)	(this)
Aveolar	Aveolar ridge and tongue tip	d, n*, l, z**, t, s**	
Palato-alveolar	Palato-aveolar boundary and tongue blade	(seizure)	ʃ (she)
Palatal	Hard palate and tongue blade	j	
Velar (soft palate)	Velum and back of tongue	g	k
Glottal	Glottis		h

* nasals ** fricatives

Fig. 60. Main classifications of consonant sounds simplified.
(International Phonetic Alphabet Symbols)

The mechanism of articulation

Patterns of everyday speech tend to be used in pop singing, however this is not so true for recital and opera. Ideally, the ease of everyday speech can be used in all singing as long as diction is not poor or careless. The person with fine speech habits will have fewer obstacles to overcome. Since one speaks more than one sings, incorrect patterns become ingrained and can only be corrected with intensely hard work. However, when these are corrected (at least for singing) the singer will be able to maintain clear diction and adequate space for resonation. It is not unusual to hear singers with good habits of articulation while singing and poor habits in their speech. The better the speech habits, the greater will be the ease of producing these sounds in singing. Typical articulatory problems which interfere with ease of singing include tension in the lips and tongue, over-active muscles controlling the lower jaw, and/or a tongue that does not function independently of the jaw to produce consonants.

Articulatory structures fall into two categories: those that are fixed, for example the teeth, and those that are movable like the tongue. Obviously the singer can do nothing about the fixed ones, however the relation of the moving parts to these will influence vocal production by altering the shape of the resonator. In his research on over-articulation of consonants, Scotto di Carlo (1979) concluded that such *"articulation has particularly disrupting effects on the beauty of vibrato, the continuity of legato, the aesthetics of attacks, sustained phrases and releases, which are generally considered to play a considerable part in the quality of singing."*

Efficient articulation demands movements of the lower jaw, tongue, lips and soft palate that are precise and without undue tension. These structures can then react easily and co-ordinate with breathing and the postural support structure. A brief discussion of the anatomy of the jaws, tongue and lips are given here to aid in understanding the complex patterns of activity used in articulation.

Anatomical aspects of articulation

Fixed structures

Fixed articulation structures have the important function of acting as a base for the action of the mobile articulators and include the teeth, the alveolar ridges supporting the teeth, and the hard palate (Figs. 46 and 61).

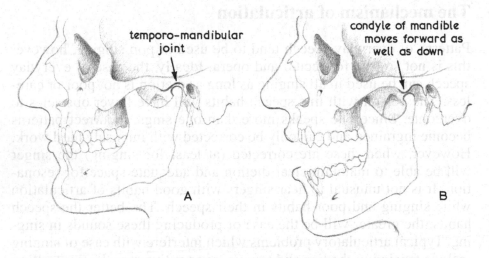

Fig. 61. Drawing of the left temporo-mandibular joint with the mouth closed *(A)* and opened *(B)*. Note the positions of the head of the mandible, particularly that it slides forward as the mouth is opened.

Movable structures

a) The mandible

The muscles controlling the mandible or lower jaw are the most powerful muscles of the head. They are used primarily in biting and chewing. In singing the muscles are balanced with other structures of the mechanism of singing to allow only that movement of the jaw which is necessary for articulation. As stated earlier, too much movement, as exhibited by singers with protrusion or a "jutting jaw", makes efficient articulation impossible.

The joint connecting the mandible to the skull is called the temporo-mandibular joint and is capable of far more complex actions than those of a simple hinge joint (Fig. 61). Even the simple opening and closing of jaws is a compound movement. Place a finger just in front of the small flap of skin in front of the ear and open your mouth, you feel the head of the mandible sliding forward, forward and downwards, as well as rotating to open up the mouth. The reverse occurs as you close. A moment's thought about its actions makes one realise that in addition to opening and closing the mouth by depression and elevation of the mandible, there are also the side-to-side motions of chewing, protraction or protrusion when the head of the mandible slides forward, and retraction when is slides backwards. The powerful muscles of mastication control these actions. While most of these actions are necessary for chewing or mastication, they are not so essential for singing, a fact that bears repeating because too often singers will blur the distinction between these actions and produce "chewed" speech and singing.

The muscles of mastication such as the masseter, temporalis and medial pterygoids, are powerful elevators of the jaw (Fig. 62). When acting together the left and right lateral pterygoid muscles and some fibres of both medical pterygoids protract the jaw, and the posterior fibres of the temporalis retract it (Fig. 62), it is therefore all too easy to poke the jaw forwards in an exaggerated fashion. Side-to-side motion is produced by alternate action of the two pterygoid muscles of opposite sides. The depressors of the mandible are few. It is thought that the initial process of depression begins with contraction of the lateral pterygoids and anterior portions of the digastrics, and that gravity and relaxation of the elevator muscles then do the rest. Some of the muscles activating the jaw can be palpated and one can observe in a mirror the various changes that occur when muscles like the temporalis and masseter contract. The pterygoids are too deep to be felt. When the mouth is opened against a closing force, a number of the suprahyoid muscles become involved. However, for singing the mouth is not opened against resistance but instead the muscles of mastication like the temporalis and pterygoids act to suspend the jaw while the masseter is relaxed.

Suspension and release of the jaw must be pursued consciously for most people because their speech patterns tend to either be careless or over articulated. Muscles like the masseter are especially sensitive to positions of the jaws and are capable of many gradations of contraction and relaxation (for example, as a test, place a hair between the teeth; it will

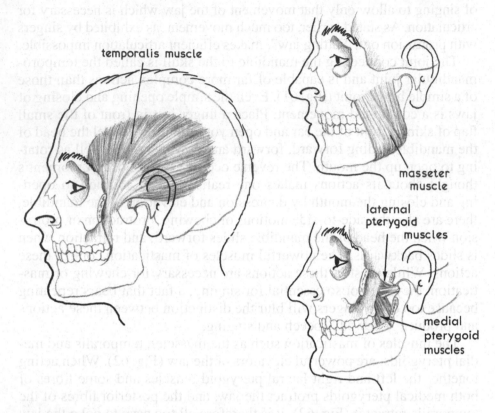

Fig. 62. Drawing of the main muscles of mastication on the left side.
Temporalis, masseter and the medial pterygoid muscles are powerful elevators of the jaw.
Action of both lateral pterygoid muscles is a prelude to opening the mouth (see Fig. 62); it
pulls the head of the mandible forwards. Symmetrical action of the left and right medial and
lateral pterygoids protrudes the jaw, and alternating action of the left right muscles produces
grinding, chewing movements.

The *temporalis* muscle is fan shaped and *arises* from the whole of the temporal fossa and
deep surface of the temporal fascia. It passes between the side of the skull and zygomatic
arch to have a strong *insertion* on the inside, top, anterior and posterior borders of the coronoid process of the mandible.

The *masseter* is quadrilateral in shape and arises in three layers from the zygomatic process
of the maxilla, deep surface of the anterior two-thirds of the zygomatic arch and the posterior
portion of its lower border. The *insertion* of the three layers is on the angle, lower, middle
and upper parts of the ramus of the mandible with a small portion of the middle layer insert-
ing on the coronoid process.

The *lateral pterygoid* has an upper head arising from the infratemporal surface and crest of
the greater wing of the sphenoid bone and a lower head *arising* from the lateral surface of
the lateral pterygoid plate. It *inserts* into a small depression on the front of the neck of the
mandible and the articular capsule and disc of the temporomandibular joint.

The *medial pterygoid* has complex *origins* including those from the medial surface of the
lateral pterygoid plate and pyramidal surface of the palatine bone and *inserts* on the lower
and back part of the medial surface of the ramus and angle of the mandible. This muscle
along with the masseter forms a sling for the mandible.

be easily felt.) These gradations enable the singer to hold or lock the jaw into a variety of positions, all detrimental to good singing. These muscles often contribute to facial expression for example when under tension the jaws are clenched. The contractions of muscles around the jaw can cause obvious deficiencies in vocal quality. This can be demonstrated readily by altering positions of the jaw while sustaining a note. Even when a singer cannot hear the difference, it is detectible by an audience.

When singers protrude the lower jaw while pronouncing consonants, the larynx is pulled forwards causing an alteration in the shape of the air passage and thereby altering tonal quality. Another problem occurs when differing degrees of muscle tension or relaxation affect the jaw causing it to shift to one side or the other. It is not unusual to see such unevenness manifested in a singer whose jaw is shifted laterally to the right or left while singing, particularly during sustained high notes. Learning to balance the jaw might seem to be a simple process however, in practice, it is not so because of firmly ingrained eating and speaking habits.

b) The lips

The importance of the lips in influencing the quality of specific sound and resonance has already been discussed and, at the risk of sounding repetitious, certain features are important to emphasise. With the tongue, their role in efficient articulation is paramount. The muscular structure of the lips is provided by a confluence of several muscles of facial expression including the buccinator. These muscles fall into five groups depicted in Fig. 65:

1. The elevators of the upper lip and corners of the mouth.
2. The orbicularis oris closes the lips and also protrudes them as its action becomes stronger.
3. The depressors of the lower lip.
4. The retractors of the corners of the mouth and lips.
5. The mentalis protrudes the lower lip for pouting.

With so many muscles and varieties of shapes of jaws and individual habits of speech and facial tensions, learning to release the lips is essential for proper articulation. It is pleasing to see and hear a singer who looks natural rather than contorted in performance. A critic once remarked about a singer: *"As an actress she has not talent for opera. Her mouth is distended in a perpetuity of a grin, which is moderated neither by affliction or death ... Yet this grin never moderates, and her enthusiastic admirers venture to affirm that she could not sing without it; if this were the case, she must at once be pronounced totally unfit for tragedy, but the idea is absurd; nothing but a lock-jaw could compel such an unnatural distortion"* (Gattey, 1979).

c) The tongue

The tongue can be either an asset or liability to the singer; undue muscular contraction will cause the tongue to change the shape of the space in the mouth and thus distort the resonances and inhibit efficient articulation. Extrinsic muscles of the tongue are attached to the mandible, styloid process, hyoid bone, soft palate and wall of the pharynx, and its movements can therefore influence the three latter structures (Fig. 64). There are also four sets of intrinsic muscles which are contained strictly within the tongue and have no bony attachments.

Those paired extrinsic muscles important to speech and singing are:

1. The genioglossus muscles form most of the bulk of the tongue and are each comprised of three main bundles of fibres, which may act together or more independently in articulation. When acting as a whole, the muscle protrudes the tongue. The anterior bundle draws the tip downwards. The middle and posterior bundles draw the middle portion of the tongue downwards.
2. The hyoglossus muscles are thin, like a postage stamp, and the fibres pass vertically upwards from the hyoid bone and mingle with others of the tongue. The muscles depress the sides of the posterior portion of the tongue.
3. The styloglossus muscles arise from the styloid process and pass along the sides of the tongue and intermingle with fibres of the hyoglossus. The contraction of these muscles causes the tongue to move upwards and backwards.
4. The palatoglossus arises from the underside of the soft palate and is inserted into the sides of the posterior part of the tongue. Its action depends on the rigidity of its attachments and the state of contraction of the intrinsic muscles of the tongue. For example, when the palate is too tense it may mean that the root of the tongue will be pulled upwards. When the intrinsic muscles of the tongue are contracted the resultant action is most likely palatal depression. The palatoglossus forms the anterior pillar of the fauces, or palatoglossal fold, which is readily observed by looking at the throat in a mirror (Fig. 65).

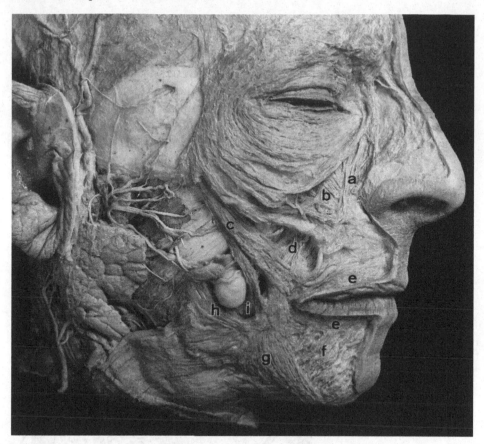

Fig. 63. The muscles of facial expression and the lips.
(By kind permission of the Anatomy Department of the Royal College of Surgeons of England.)
The muscles influencing different movements of the lips include:
1. Elevation of upper lip and corner of the mouth
   Levator labii superioris alaeque nasi *(a)*
   Levator labii superioris *(b)*
   Zygomaticus major and minor *(c)*
   Levator anguli oris *(d)*
2. Closure and protrusion of the lip
   Orbicularis oris *(e)*
3. Depression of the lower lip
   Depressor labii inferioris *(f)*
   Depressor anguli oris *(g)*
4. Retraction of the corners of the mouth and lips
   Risorius *(h)*
   Buccinator *(i)*
5. Protrusion of lower lip
   Mentalis (not shown)

There are four paired sets of intrinsic muscles of the tongue; these are superior and inferior longitudinal fibres, transverse and vertical ones (Fig. 65). The fibres course among the fibres of other extrinsic muscles and their actions alter the shape of the tongue. The superior and inferior longitudinal muscles tend to shorten and broaden the shape of the tongue, the superior ones also turn up the tip and sides to make the upper surface convex. The transverse muscle fibres narrow and thicken the tongue. The vertical fibres flatten and broaden it.

The ability to alter the concavity or convexity of the tongue is thought to be inherited and not all singers can achieve the much-talked-about longitudinal "grooved tongue". Conscious efforts to do this in a person

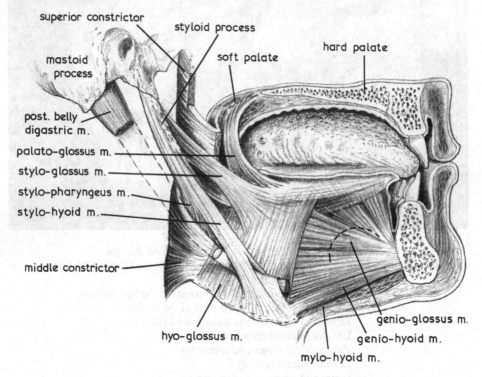

Fig. 64. The extrinsic muscles of the tongue seen from the right. (The hard palate and mandible have been cut in half).

The paired *genio-glossus* muscle has fibers which arise from two small protuberances, the genial tubercles, on the inside of the mandible, and spread out like fans. These fibers form three main bundles: anterior, middle and posterior.

Each *hyo-glossus* muscle arises in a line from the greater horns and outer half of the body of the hyoid bone. The fibers pass vertically upwards and mingle with others of the tongue.

Each *stylo-glossus* muscle arises from the styloid process near the apex, passes downwards and forwards and divides in two portions; a longitudinal one which is inserted in front of the hyo-glossus, and oblique fibers which overlap the hyo-glossus and intermingle with its fibers.

Each palato-glossus muscle arises from the inferior portion of the soft palate and is inserted into the sides of the posterior parts of the tongue.

without the ability will produce a rigid tongue. When the singer tries consciously to form this groove intrinsic and extrinsic muscles begin to contract and the system of interconnection will cause the soft palate to move downwards and the larynx to move upward, thus limiting the available resonating spaces.

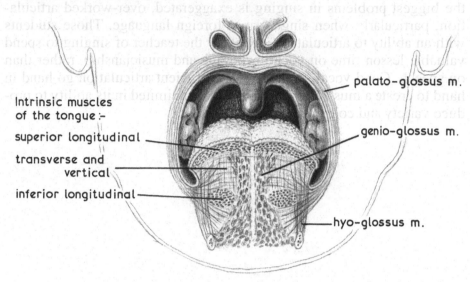

Intrinsic muscles
of the tongue :-

superior longitudinal

transverse and
vertical

inferior longitudinal

palato-glossus m.

genio-glossus m.

hyo-glossus m.

Fig. 65. Intrinsic muscles of the tongue and pillars of the fauces.
(The anterior portion of the tongue has been removed)

Summary

Spontaneous, free symmetrical articulation created by efficiency of the muscles associated with articulation in co-ordination with the remainder of the structures used in singing will contribute enormously to meaning, style, tonal clarity and quality. As a result the face of the singer will be able to look natural and respond easily to the mood and ideas reflected in the text. The desired expression and interpretation is lost or obscured when the singer has difficulties with the technicalities of articulation. Boring though it may seem, it is one aspect of performance that can be practised assiduously. When the tongue and mandible do not move properly, practice and teaching can cure the bad habit. Patience and a mirror are indispensable in learning good habits of diction.

Singers everywhere would benefit from meticulous attention being given to the free and balanced movement of the jaw and release of tension from the lips. The result will be an articulation that is amazingly clear, an easily produced sound by the singer and understanding of the text by the audience.

Singers who are taught proper pronunciation and articulation in their native speech will more readily learn the diction of other languages and be better prepared to absorb the proper articulation for singing. One of the biggest problems in singing is exaggerated, over-worked articulation, particularly when singing in a foreign language. Those students with an ability to articulate freely allow the teacher of singing to spend valuable lesson time on vocal technique and musicianship, rather than on speech. Good vocal production and efficient articulation go hand in hand to create a musical instrument that is unlimited in its ability to produce variety and color.

Vocal health 10

Speech is such a vital and immediate means of communication that when it is lost, the best of substitutes is found severely wanting, for loss and/or damage to the larynx and absence of powers of vocalisation are major deprivations, even tragedies. Informed singers are acutely aware of the need to prevent vocal damage, however many potential singers are uninformed and unfortunately early warnings are so insidious that they are often overlooked. Hoarseness, even in the absence of discomfort, is nature's signal to rest the voice, yet unwisely most people tend to force it to function despite this sign of overwork.

At one time or another everyone suffers from some form of vocal disorder, and for singers this may jeopardise a career and thereafter a livelihood. Since many serious problems arise because of ignorance and lack of care on the part of the singer, a discussion of general health is in order before the specific problems are broached.

General health and nutrition

The physical demands on a singer can be very great when one considers the energy needed in performance as well as the wearing lifestyle inherent in the profession. Because the body is the singer's instrument, it behoves him to stay in good health with proper rest, sensible diet and regular physical conditioning.

Singers and actors who have full days and late rehearsals are often unaware that a tired body means a tired voice. To perform under these circumstances is unfair to the audience and potentially harmful to the performer. Individuals differ considerably in the number of hours needed for refreshing sleep, so it is of no value to suggest a precise requirement here. Each performer must judge how he or she feels day after day, whether there is the energy necessary for a fine performance or a beneficial practice, and tailor the pattern of sleep accordingly.

Stories abound about the eating habits of famous singers; however the sensible pursuit of good health is governed by a few simple rules.

- There needs to be adequate protein in the diet, to combat wear and tear of tissues. It is obtained from many different foods – meat, eggs, cheese, milk, and for those who never take animal protein there are various types of pulses[1].
- In addition to protein, everyone needs carbohydrates and fat in their diet. Fad diets, which stress one type of food for periods of time, tend to create huge losses of energy as weight is lost.
- The sensible diet is a balanced one combined with adequate physical exercise that maintains good nutrition with the proper vitamins and minerals present for good health and vitality.

In general, obese singers are not in fashion today. In the past it was thought that fat contributed to resonance. This fallacy arose because singers who lost weight too quickly by virtually starving themselves, lost both physical and vocal energy, and the loss of fat rather than energy was falsely blamed for the decreased vocal quality. The performer who needs to lose weight must do so slowly over a long period of time lest he suffers from detrimental fatigue and lack of energy that diminish performance. Today (with very few notable exceptions), opera companies prefer singers who sing well and look convincing on stage; and the overweight prima donna who sings rooted to the spot while the rest of the company interprets the libretto, is no longer acceptable. A young overweight singer is not likely to be engaged, and even a singer with a very special voice may only be given a contract subject to loss of weight.

The third factor, the need for physical fitness, understandably tends to be over-looked by performers who are subjected to long hours of practice and rehearsal. Physical activity involving free movement and increased depth of breathing is valuable to any healthy person. Dancing, jogging, walking, callisthenics, tennis, swimming and stretching exercises are particularly helpful. Swimming is a valuable exercise for the whole body, which is buoyed up by the water; however singers would be best advised to refrain from diving and underwater swimming because of risks of nasal congestion and possible ear trouble. Weightlifting could be detrimental because it tends to overdevelop the muscles of the

---

[1] Those vegetarians who eat no animal protein must carefully analyze the protein they do eat, so that they get a complete range of necessary protein containing all essential amino acids.

neck and the adductors of the vocal folds. When closed the latter increase intra-thoracic pressure used to support the spine during initial phases of heavy lifting.

A body that responds well physically gives a sense of wellbeing and energy and is therefore more responsive for vocal performance. Physical wellbeing, mental, emotional, and psychological stability go hand in hand, and when one sleeps and eats well and is physically fit, then generally the emotional attitude is good. The singer plagued with problems tends to ignore his physical wellbeing and thus adversely affects his stage work. Inevitably singers like the rest of the world, have problems, and audiences are notoriously intolerant of shortcomings whatever the source. The wise singer understands that when problems arise they must be handled in a mature, logical way rather than being allowed to trigger mental depression and physical deterioration. Söderström (1979), a Swedish singer of international reputation, carries this one step further by stating:

"If one is to survive such a life as ours, one must learn one very important thing …. to be able to be alone with yourself. Whether you are nervous, happy or unhappy, there will be many moments in your life when you cannot share your feelings with anyone else, when you are alone with no one else but yourself and your sensitive little instrument, and you wait endlessly long hours before at last it is time to go to the place where your audience is assembled. Then it is a question of being able to live with yourself and knowing how to occupy yourself to keep you mental balance. Good nerves and mental balance … yes, they are often necessary as you go through the mill as a singer. The mere fact that everything you do will be judged publicly, in itself takes some getting used to …"

Even with a diligent health regimen vocal problems may occur, and the singer needs to learn to distinguish between serious and minor issues.

Hoarseness

One of the first symptoms of abnormal vocal production is hoarseness, which gives a breathy, rasping, rough, quality to the voice. It is caused by some change in the edges of the vocal folds which allow excess air to escape, and it *must never* be considered a normal condition. It can be caused by something as simple and transient as a cold or allergy or, more serious, there may be a local disorder in the larynx or some abnormal pressure on the motor nerves to the intrinsic muscles of the larynx. Hoarseness that lasts more than about ten days requires prompt investigation. The healthy voice is clear, and one that has been hoarse for a long period of time indicates neglect rather than a norm for that voice. The brief discussion which follows will deal with conditions most likely to affect singers.

a) Allergies

Allergies can cause swelling of the tissues in the throat and larynx leading to hoarseness. Airborne irritants like pollen, dust, toxic substances and cigarette smoke make a singer's life particularly miserable. When allergic reactions occur frequently enough to keep the singer out of performance, even for thirty per cent of the time, another profession might be well advised, for it is impossible to retain professional credibility in such circumstances. However, many of these allergies can be brought under control especially when professional health advice is sought early and followed faithfully.

b) Respiratory disease

The most frequent respiratory disease is the common cold, heralded by sneezing, sniffling or coughing. However, these symptoms are sometimes the prelude to more serious infections of the sinuses, and even acute bronchitis or pneumonia. Unless heavy and febrile, a cold usually does not hamper the singer. Even with mild symptoms, increase fluid intake and rest, and when soreness in the throat supervenes, singing must be limited.

Clearly with a severe cold all singing must cease. Singing with a voice made hoarse by swollen mucous membranes has produced many vocal cripples by leading to chronic hoarseness. There are some standard rules for the singer with a cold:

1. Get plenty of rest
2. Speak as little as possible. Do not sing when you can possibly avoid doing so.
3. Drink plenty of fluids (*not alcohol* this induces even more swelling of nasal mucous membranes). They help to reduce fever and make the mucous secretions thinner.
4. Dryness increases discomfort so keep the throat moist by sucking a lozenge or pastille. It does not matter whether the lozenge is medicated.

5. When a decongestant is needed, ask for one that does not dry the mucous membranes of the nose and throat. These are readily available and a great many popular over-the-counter preparations are not good for singers because their drying effect increases irritation of the lining of the vocal tract.

6. Avoid vigorous clearing of the throat and violent coughing. While it is necessary to empty the lungs of foreign material, such explosive action is extremely hard on the vocal folds and can cause hoarseness to linger for weeks after the other symptoms have subsided. A better way to clear the lungs is by inhaling steam. The airborne steam will filter to levels below the vocal folds where it can moisten and loosen some of the hardened secretions of the trachea and bronchi. In some countries a way of treating congested lungs is by means of postural drainage and physiotherapy which aid the upward movement of excess fluid and mucous.

7. Make good use of vocally inactive time to memorise music and texts. Listen to records of your repertoire as sung by various artists.

8. *Be considerate enough to keep your distance from fellow singers. They do not want to share your disease, which is spread by airborne droplets.*

How can one determine when typical cold symptoms are actually symptoms of a more serious illness? Normally the mucous secretions of an early cold are clear, with secondary bacterial infection they become greenish, grey or yellow pus. When this characteristic is noticed, it is best for the singer to consult a professional health practitioner. A bacterial infection treated properly can be alleviated rapidly, but when neglected or inadequately treated, it can become a chronic problem. In the early stages of any respiratory disease, including a cold or sinusitis, it is best to stay indoors, in as even a temperature as possible and to take plenty of fluids and vitamins such as A, B and C (A is particularly recommended for health of the mucous membranes, B for stress and C for healing).

c) Vocal misuse

A singer practising for several hours a day can induce oedema (swelling) of the vocal folds from overuse and friction. Some light hoarseness may occur immediately after rehearsal, and with rest it will probably be gone by the next day. However, when hoarseness occurs after every practice, or when it does not become clear by the next day, it is an indication the voice is either being improperly used or that there may be something more seriously amiss. Usually it implies that the singer is doing one of two things: over-blowing, thus putting excessive air pressure on the vocal folds, or using too much muscular effort in the larynx to produce the sound. While these faults will cause chronic hoarseness in the short run, the long-range effect of such faulty vocal technique can lead to more serious difficulties such as development of vocal nodules, polyps, chronic hoarseness or muscular fatigue (Figs. 66 and 67).

Vocal nodules and polyps are more common in pop and rock singers and in salesmen and preachers because they rely on stress and tension

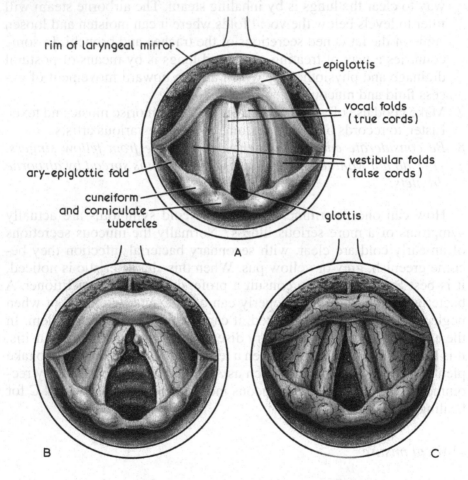

Fig. 66. Normal and pathological vocal folds.
A is a drawing of normal vocal folds during speech. In this drawing there is a chink between the arytenoid cartilages so the sound is probably breathy in quality.
B shows irregular nodules on the edges of the anterior parts of each vocal fold, also the engorgement of the fine vessels.
C depicts acute inflammation of the larynx with marked swelling and engorgement of vessels on the epiglottis, ary-epiglottic folds, and on the vestibular and vocal folds.

in the production of sound. They are the result of speaking and singing habits that cause too much friction when the vocal folds vibrate thus causing irritation of the edges of the folds.

Nodules generally begin as a haematoma or bruise on the edges of the folds and the symptom is hoarseness. When this haematoma is ignored it enlarges and eventually develops either into a hard or soft nodule or a polyp, which is a nodule with a stalk. When such a lesion is small, vocal rest and proper technique may allow it to slowly disappear. When large, it requires surgical removal, a simple procedure with the sophisticated techniques currently available. *However,* once the lesion is removed, voice therapy is imperative because when the singer (or speaker) returns to the same patterns of vocal production, the growth will return. Surgery only eliminates the symptom; it does not cure the causal bad habit.

Singers most commonly affected are those who must perform in clubs and cabaret. Their vocal techniques more often resemble yelling than true singing, and they sing long hours in noisy smoke-filled rooms. The entire situation is antithetical to good singing and many a club singer must weigh the advantages of earning a good salary for a few years against the possibility of ruining his voice for life. The saddest cases include the many singers who never succeed in their career and have ruined their voices in the attempt.

Laryngitis is the inflammation of the tissues of the larynx and can be brought about by an infection, allergies, yelling, talking, or singing improperly or for too long. Since chronic laryngitis may be an indication of past or probably continuing abuse of the vocal folds, it is logical to rest the voice until the symptoms have disappeared. However since speaking is such an important function in one's life, most people continue to talk or whisper, thus further straining the vocal folds. When acute or chronic laryngitis strikes, silence is required, no whispering even, and when this warning is persistently ignored physical changes are likely to occur in the vocal folds.

Muscular fatigue is the most difficult condition to detect or remedy and usually occurs in people who have pressured their voices over a long period of time – even years. This can happen so gradually that the performer is completely unaware of it. The first signs are hoarseness or a wobbling sound indicative of improper function of vocal muscles which have had more strain than they can take. When the misuse has been long and intense, bowing of the vocal folds can occur. Just as an athlete's muscles will not respond when they are over used the singer's vocal muscles will also rebel. The difference is that the singer does not always "get the message" and continues to vocalise under stress. Sometimes the voice just stops working overnight, and the uninformed singer will be unable to comprehend the fact that the sudden failure of his voice actually came about after months, probably years of continuous abuse. The prognosis for restoring this type of battered vocal folds to normal function is not a good one.

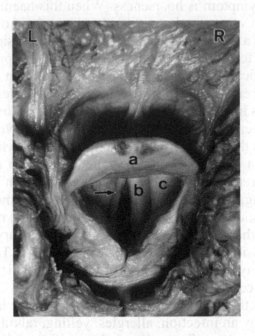

Fig. 67. Abnormal right vocal fold.
(By kind permission of the Anatomy Department of the Royal College of Surgeons of England.) Dissection of human larynx showing ulceration on the epiglottis *(a)*, irregularity of the left (↑), and gross thickening of the right vocal *(b)* and vestibular folds *(c)*. (No medical history was available.)

d) Hoarseness of psychogenic origin

The term psychogenic is often used to refer to those vocal problems for which there is alteration of the sound, yet there is no observable change in the vocal folds. Sometimes hysterical hoarseness may present itself when a singer is under great stress. All singers experience some form of stage fright, particularly the inexperienced. However, intensity of purpose and solid understanding of what they are doing will usually dispel that fright without damage to performance. Very occasionally the singer may become so frightened that acute hoarseness will appear on the day before or the day of a performance. It is difficult for the teacher to ascertain whether or not the problem is psychogenic in origin. Often by talking to the singer and boosting his confidence the problem will disappear.

At other times more is required. For example when the singer can cough or clear his throat with a clear sound, the problem is unlikely to be an organic one. Getting the singer to laugh or cough and pointing out that he has managed to clear his voice may help. Failing this, the laryngologist often can be a calming influence by seeing the singer, offering advice and even administering medication when he feels it is necessary.

Now there is much more interest in the stress related to performance by teachers and health professionals. One of the most potent ways of alleviating stress is by making sure the teaching studio has a positive and supportive environment. (See Chapter 3). The psychological makeup of the performer is complex and a great deal of nourishment is needed in the process of learning and performing.

Drugs

Singers need to be made aware that any drug inhaled, swallowed, or injected may affect the muscles and tissues needed for vocal production. Habit-forming and exceedingly dangerous drugs like heroin, cocaine, crack, and even marijuana and salvia, and some of those commonly prescribed alter emotional sensitivity. Since a sensitive performance demands all one's faculties to be at their keenest, in the long run a drug addiction dooms a singer to failure. The performer influenced by drugs may perceive his tone as a freer one at the very moment that the actual sound heard by the audience may be garbled and lacking in quality and control.

Sometimes before a performance a singer will take a tranquilliser or muscle relaxant to "calm his nerves". Unfortunately such drugs may relax the laryngeal muscles, and one can only speculate whether the performance will simply be comfortable or so relaxed that the singing is off-key.

Alcohol is no exception; a number of notable singers have required an alcoholic bracer before going on stage, and while they may have found the practice helpful, it cannot be recommended *carte blanche*. The habitual use of alcohol can pose serious problems and affect the voice in number of ways. Since alcohol acts as a muscle relaxant and depressant much like a tranquilliser, the control of the vocal folds and sensitivity of the throat may be impaired. In addition alcohol has a drying effect on the tissues of the vocal tract and in time can cause irritation evidenced by the typically raspy or hoarse voice of the chronic drinker.

To put it quite simply, any of the above drugs is capable of causing the performer to have a lower critical appraisal and more tolerant judgement of personal performance at a time when these faculties need to be at their sharpest. The performance is more reliable when the singer can use his own inner resources, confidence and technique to allow emotions to flow freely.

Smoking

For the singer there need not be a dilemma – smoking is detrimental to vocal health. The first effect that smoking has on the body is to dry the mucous membranes that line the vocal folds, larynx and trachea. Without the needed moisture the vocal folds do not function as well and the singer's sense of feel of what is happening is diminished. A far more devastating effect is the damage done by the toxic elements of smoke to the cells of the respiratory tract. The cells below the glottis have hair-like projections (cilia). These cilia beat upward to propel foreign matter from the bronchial tree and trachea. Smoke impairs the ciliary function and in severe cases may kill the ciliated cells over a period of time. Toxic substances can then become embedded in the respiratory tract where eventually they may affect the lungs and/or larynx, sometimes leading to the formation of a tumour or growth. When this happens, a singer's career and perhaps even his life will be endangered. Current reports state that smoking is one of the causes of lung cancer and that there are connection between smoking and other cancers of the respiratory tract and between smoking and heart disease.

Special vocal problems of women

The menstrual cycle can affect the voices in some women. There is no consistent pattern in an individual from month to month, however the general pre-menstrual build up of fluid can affect the vocal folds so that they swell, and the voice sounds tired or hoarse and has diminished power and flexibility. Under these circumstances it is best not to force the voice, and a singer with severe symptoms is advised to abstain from performing for one to three days during that time. European opera companies are much more helpful than their American counterparts because they excuse the women from performing during particularly difficult days.

The effects of the contraceptive pill and other hormones have been of increasing interest to laryngologists and research workers. Damsté (1964) and many more recent studies have found that these drugs can have virilizing effects on the voice. Some young women using oral contraceptives have experienced changes leading to masculinization with deepening and roughening of vocal quality. Evidence suggests that for pubescent girls and young women these changes are not reversed even when the drugs are withdrawn. Singers in their teens and twenties are advised to search for other means of contraception.

The use of anabolic drugs (steroids) and hormones by menopausal women has also been strongly criticised for causing changes of voice.

Surgical procedures pertinent to singers

Everyone tends to be apprehensive about undergoing surgery and a conscientious doctor makes every effort to allay fears by explaining both the problem and the corrective procedure to his patient. A patient is expected to ask questions until he is reassured about any operation that has been prescribed; and a singer must feel free to express concern about the effect of proposed surgery on his performance.

The surgical procedures most likely to affect the voice are bronchoscopy, removal of benign or malignant growths, tonsillectomy and thyroidectomy, or general anaesthesia administered by passing a tube through the glottis into the trachea. Prolonged surgery using intubation can irritate and damage the edges of the vocal folds and those physicians sensitive to the needs of singers are looking for more suitable techniques. Singers are rightly concerned and should discuss the necessity of intubation with the anaesthetist. In general it is considered the safest way to administer and control general anaesthesia, and a singer might find it difficult to persuade an anaesthetist convinced of its need to follow another course. When recovering from the anaesthesia, it is usual to find that the premedication, gasses and drugs have made the throat uncomfortably dry. This problem lasts for a few hours. Once back in the room and fully conscious one can ask for a lozenge or pastille to help alleviate the dryness. A vaporiser is the most helpful way to alleviate the discomfort and it is worth requesting one.

Bronchoscopy is a means of looking directly at a patient's vocal folds, trachea and air passages while he is sedated and probably under general anaesthesia. This procedure is usually followed when some serious and possibly deeply placed trouble is suspected and cannot be visualised during the office visit, or when the patient is too nervous to allow adequate visualisation of the vocal folds any other way.

The advent of micro and laser surgery has made removal of benign growths of the vocal folds a relatively simple task. Doctors are able to remove tissue by the millimetre or less without leaving noticeable scar tissue to impair the quality of vocal production. However, even after such surgery, the patient must remain on total vocal rest throughout the healing process, and when the tissues are healed, voice therapy is advised in order to correct the vocal misuse that caused the nodules in the first place.

The tonsils occupy the space between the anterior and posterior pillars of the fauces (overlying the palatoglossus and palatopharyngeus muscles, Fig. 65). When they are infected and swell, they take up a large space in the oral pharynx. Constant infection and quinsy (abscesses) are indications for tonsillectomy. There is no anatomical connection between the tonsils and the larynx and singers can rest assured that the removal of two, large, infected, swollen and sound absorbing lumps (tonsils) in the throat will probably enhance vocal quality by making more space available and removing a source of recurrent infection. Post-operatively the singer will be aware of two new sensations. First, the scar tissue will be stiff for some time, making it more difficult to elevate the soft palate. However, the difficulty is not serious, unless the singer is too reluctant to stretch this scar tissue. When this is so, the palate may well remain low during phonation, air will escape through the nose, and a nasal tone will be produced. The second sensation is due to the additional space in the throat, and therefore the singer has to adapt to the inevitable changes in his perceptions. As long as the singer and his teacher have a clear picture of what happens during and after tonsillectomy, it does not have be a worrying experience.

Any surgery in the area of the neck and in the face where the facial nerve (seventh cranial nerve) is located can pose a potentially serious problem. The facial nerve is responsible for the motor supply of muscles of facial expression, and severe damage to this nerve leads to loss of all movements and expression on the affected side. Closure of the eyelids is impossible, and the mouth is pulled towards the opposite side by the active muscles. Facial expression, so necessary for effective singing, is not only impaired, it also looks unsightly. The sound and articulation are affected because the lips and cheeks are distorted in speaking and singing.

In some rare instances a singer may need thyroid surgery. In expert hands this carries a remote element of risk, because the branching of the recurrent laryngeal nerve and its relationship with the inferior thyroid artery vary considerably. This nerve is the motor nerve to the intrinsic muscles of the larynx and when the nerve is irritated, the symptoms of hoarseness or vocal fold paralysis may appear. However, when this nerve is cut, permanent paralysis of the vocal fold results and singing professionally will be out of the question. Any singer for whom thyroid surgery has been advised needs to have a thorough discussion of the possible effects, and only undergo the operation at the hands of an acknowledged expert. Although the hazard is very small indeed, it is dishonest to guarantee a 100% recovery to every single patient.

Singers and their doctors

Physicians who see many singers in their practice know that the singers are sensitive and their vocal folds are like the muscles of a trained athlete. They are therefore sympathetic to seemingly minor transient problems, while other throat specialists who are not used to treating singers may be insensitive to their needs, especially when they are compared with more acute diseases. While singers' vocal difficulties may seem less significant than some life-threatening pathologies, the aware health professional realises that even the slightest change noticed by the singer may be serious enough to endanger his livelihood.

In some cases when singers and doctors have problems in communicating with one another, the singer becomes suspicious and the doctor intolerant. The singer who goes to the laryngologist with a certain amount of apprehension will be in a better position when he knows what the examination entails and comes prepared to give a precise account of specific symptoms to the doctor. Before examining the patient a doctor always elicits a history. It helps the doctor when the singer brings a carefully prepared account to his complaint. The singer can be most useful to the physician by describing his symptoms without using sign language and singer's jargon. Listening carefully and answering each point accurately will help to avoid misleading the doctor and wasting time. It is important to tell the physician where there is pain, whether that pain is dull and aching or sharp, whether it hurts to swallow or breathe, how long these symptoms have lasted, and any unusual aspect of his singing or practice that may have affected vocal production. After taking a history, the doctor will look at the vocal folds by holding an angled laryngeal mirror on the soft palate or by means of fibre optic and stroboscopic tools. The examination is awkward rather than painful, and requires the singer to have enough will power to relax the lower jaw and tongue. While using a piece of gauze or other material to hold the tongue out, the doctor will ask his patient to sing or say /i/ (as in meet), an almost impossible feat with the tongue in such a position. However, it is by this method that the physician obtains the best view of the movements of the vocal folds.

A good physician never prescribes medication for symptoms like hoarseness without first determining the underlying cause. When a performer has created vocal difficulties through the misuse of his voice, medication may eliminate the swelling or symptoms temporarily, however the real problem of vocal abuse will only be prolonged. On the other hand, singers with colds who are obliged to see that the show goes on, may require the immediate help of a laryngologist to assure that the curtain will go up. Even then, with serious symptoms in evidence the performer and the physician must decide whether that one performance is worth risking problems that may follow from singing under adverse conditions. The singer may well have to choose between cancelling one performance in order to prevent many future cancellations.

Complementary health professionals available to singers

Today singers have many options when they seek help with their concerns about physical and emotional problems. In addition to the allopathic medical profession there exists a wide variety of nutritionists, speech and voice therapists, osteopaths, cranial-sacral therapists, various Eastern and Western massage techniques, body balancing and applied kinesiology techniques, many types of psychological counselling and numerous other therapies.

New healing techniques developed from both Eastern and Western sources are proving to have profound effects on the body/mind relationship. Quantum Touch™ and EFT™ (Emotional Freedom Technique) are two types of energy healing used by doctors, psychologists, alternative healers, and families. Quantum Touch™ includes use of the hands, mind, sending energy, and breathing as bases for healing. EFT™ uses a combination of affirmations and tapping on the ends of acupuncture meridians as its basis. Qigong, acupuncture, ayurvedic techniques are just a few of the popular Eastern based techniques that have proved beneficial to many. Professional singers often seek the help of complementary practitioners to ensure that they are caring for their general fitness and wellbeing, and they are taking personal responsibility for preventing serious problems.

Care of the voice

The foregoing discussion has touched on a few specific vocal problems, because it is of primary importance for the singer to know what can be done on a day-to-day basis to prevent trouble. While good health, proper nutrition and fitness will help to ward off viruses and bacterial infections, it is almost impossible to avoid getting a respiratory infection at some time. The story is told of a famous singer who received a frantic call to replace a colleague in a major operatic role in a distant city that evening. A flight was obtained and the singer, rather than submitting his throat to the smoke-filled airplane cabin went instead into the lavatory and locked himself in until the plane arrived at its destination. All singers do not have to lock themselves away, however they must protect themselves not only from infections but also from potential irritants like extremes in room temperatures, air conditioning, draughty concert and rehearsal halls, and smoke-filled rooms. This means avoiding social gatherings the evening before a performance, wearing proper clothing, and compensating for the drying nature of modern heating and air conditioning units by installing a humidifier or vaporiser in one's bedroom. When neither of these is available, a dish of water placed on the radiator or windowsill will help to alleviate the dryness.

Some singers develop the bad habit of clearing their throats. This is a self-conscious gesture which, when allowed to continue, becomes a habit difficult to break. No matter how insistent the urge to clear becomes, the singer must resist because this action causes the vocal folds to come together in a rather violent manner. The resulting friction causes wear and tear on those structures and it can lead to damage. When it is really necessary to clear the throat it should be done gently with a feeling of an open throat to spare the vocal folds any undue irritation.

Finally, any discussion of care of the voice requires some words about the habits of practice. The proper use of practice time is of utmost importance and will vary accordingly to the skill and vocal strength of the performer. It is advisable for young singers who have little concept of vocal production to sing only fifteen to twenty minutes at a time, and stringently follow the regimen set by their teacher. Under ideal circumstances, two or three short practice periods can be spread over the course of a day. These short vocally active sessions may be fleshed out by thoughtful consideration of technique, studying rhythm, texts and by translating those in a foreign language and memorising. A short period of carefully planned practice, rather than the endless and repetitious singing of assigned songs, keeps the voice healthy and promotes consistent improvement of vocal technique.

The professional's problems are more involved because his/her personal schedule of practice is complicated by rehearsals called by managers producers and conductors who are all vying for his/her time. Two hours of actual singing time is enough for anyone because on a daily basis that limit will avoid vocal fatigue. With accumulated experience, the more efficient practice, learning techniques and rehearsal time will become. Singers with heavy performing commitments go through a light vocal practice, look over music and text, and then remain quiet until they warm up for the actual performance.

It is regrettable that some conductors with little working knowledge of vocal production will require singers to rehearse for long tiring hours. This is difficult for seasoned professional singers and an almost impossible situation for the novice. Even worse, are the choral conductors whose all day workshops or long rehearsals constitute the most flagrant violations of proper usage of the voice. Under such marathon conditions, the singer can never perform at his best and is usually unable to sing for days afterwards.

Poor technique is the most serious contributor to vocal difficulties, and the constant scrutiny of a good coach or teacher can avoid the psychological trauma endured by insecure singers. Greene (1924) has summed it up by saying:

"Finally, the singer should bear in mind that he is not the best judge of his own technique and that technique can never be left alone. The physical part of his work should from time to time be submitted to other inspection. No matter how high he may stand in his art, his technique is bound occasionally to grow rusty or get out of control. In such cases he will do well to submit it to a master whom he can trust."

Research in singing 11

"Finally, we admit that the science is far behind the art ... our knowledge of the vocal mechanism in singing is quite limited. There are two major bottlenecks: limitation in subjects and limitation in techniques ... Close co-operation among different disciplines is clearly essential if we are ever to solve the mysteries of the singing voice". (Hirano 1988) Twenty years later, this quote remains true. It is not easy to study an instrument that lives inside a human body.

At this time techniques and tools available to voice scientists are improving. Some of the most significant advances have been the establishment of laboratories where speech and voice scientists work hand in hand with singers and doctors to produce more research and case histories. These laboratories have contributed to positive changes in the relationship of performance and medicine are beginning to create a statistically significant body of research. This research has developed into three main streams: acoustic studies such as laryngeal vibration efficiency and vocal tract resonances, clinical medical studies, and whole body approaches using concepts taken from Body Mapping™ and Alexander technique.

While research in the last fifty years has contributed a considerable amount of information about the functional processes involved in singing, very few articles and papers cite using statistically significant numbers of subjects. Researchers often avoid criticism by calling these published findings exploratory studies and sadly, they often find their way into the literature as absolute proof. Significant advances in technology in X-ray and acoustic equipment have given us more refined avenues for studying singers. The advent of fiberoptics has revolutionized the ease with which we can see the vocal folds in action. Magnetic Resonance Imaging offers real possibilities, however it is very expensive to use. Stroboscopes have improved in quality, as have sonographs, glottographs and other acoustic equipment. Computer technology offers a myriad of possibilities from models of the larynx to new means of diagnosing problems.

However, singing is a whole body/mind and energy field endeavor and we must begin to look to many more diverse areas of research that will aid in the quest for vocal excellence and performing in the public arena. *"Often we mistake knowledge for truth and forget that the sun shines on truth from different directions and casts a different shadow each time ... Our understanding must shine from ever-new directions."* (Ristad, 1982)

As more comprehensive approaches to teaching and research on singing evolve we need to explore questions relating to the dynamic muscular balances needed throughout the body for singing. These include: how balance or lack of balance affect the functioning of the larynx, pharynx, jaw, diaphragm, etc.; and the natural and spontaneous reflex actions of the body that produce the easiest, most beautiful and healthiest sounds. The study of the biomechanics of the body during singing has been largely ignored, compared to the huge amount of research, training, and equipment devoted to biomechanics by coaches and trainers of athletes.

Trainers of modern athletes monitor performance by using high tech equipment and biometric bodysuits with embedded sensors to enable detailed analysis of movement, balance, efficiency, and health for athletic performance. Sports scientists have looked at physical alignment and efficiency (biomechanical analysis) for a variety of different sports. It is time for singers and voice scientists to look to sports research for what they can borrow in the way of techniques; much can be gained in that area. Too many of our singers are losing out by using vocal techniques that are outdated and physically inefficient. It is well known that posture affects the shape of the vocal tract, breathing patterns, energy, and image, and yet little has been done to determine effective alignment for singing. Popular television singing contests and reality shows today provide good examples of singers demonstrating physical inefficiency. Singers who can perform well in spite of this are extremely lucky.

New areas of potential research in singing

Energy work subjects such as, Brain-Gym™ (Educational kinesiology), EFT[5] (Emotional Freedom Technique), are providing great improvement for many performers, and yet little has been done to document their effects on singing. The 'timeless arts' such as Qigong, Tai chi, Yoga, and Meditation are popular and effective techniques for centering and learning to work in the *zone*.

A few teachers of singing teach Brain-Gym™ to their students with excellent results. Brain-gym relies on body feedback, simple exercises and muscles testing to help balance the right and left sides of the brain.

Artists learn, think, perform, and react in a balanced way with less interference from nerves and poor habits.

EFT™ uses affirmations in combination with tapping on the end points of selected acupuncture meridians to great effect. NLP (Neuro-linguistic-programming) is one of the most important areas of sports psychology and mind/body focusing. It is used in every area, from sport to business, where optimal performance is important.

The timeless arts are those techniques and Eastern arts such as Tai chi and Qigong (derived from martial arts) that take us into the present moment. Yoga, meditation, and spiritual work were originally parts of these systems. Alexander technique and Feldenkrais[15] are Western practices bringing the body and mind into focus or "at one" to create efficient physical and mental balance and functioning.

Techniques like the above, taken from Eastern and Western sources involve remaining totally in the present moment and living in a timeless state of being. They enable the performer to practice and perform without the constant analytical or critical mind chatter that stops spontaneity, creativity and intuition. The state of living in the Now or being timeless is what gives a performer the ability to get the job done without added tension. It enables the highest level of attainment without undue stress on the human physical and emotional systems.

Note: These arts are to be experienced because verbal descriptions cannot convey their essence. These are not intellectual pursuits. They involve being in touch with the body without interference from the intellect and the internal conversations that fill much of our time. Reading about them, or having one session, is not enough to form any kind of understanding of the experience. They bring us into the present where there is no analytical thinking or planning, but simply being fully engaged in the "now".

The limitations of our current research

Our current avenues for studying singers are limited in a number of ways:

- Scientific techniques and equipment are often uncomfortable for singers and they are wary of being research subjects (many might consider some of the electromyography done by Vennard (1971) and others heroic for singers).
- Courses in voice science, whether they are vocal anatomy, vocology, or acoustics, do not complete the picture. We need to look at the ways teachers, doctors, therapists and researchers service the world of singing.

- Current research in singing is over balanced towards acoustics and vocal fold movement, and some respiratory function analysis, with a small portion devoted to the anatomy and physiology.
- The bulk of the research has been directed at the larynx, vowels and consonants because these were easier (?) to study.
- Singers who are chosen for research studies vary considerably in their abilities and techniques, which can mean the statistics we see are a norm of idiosyncrasies rather than those of optimum vocal production. (See Appendix A for a way of classifying singers for research).
- We lack enough 'ideal' voices and bodies to produce good models for study.
- Some are concerned about losing the "mystery" of the voice by looking at it too closely.
- Empirical studies often depend on the judgment of panels of professionals in the field who often have come from diverse backgrounds and tastes and can yield a variety of results.
- There is a developing polarity between the intellectual, analytical/critical, thinking and the holistic and whole body approaches to an art that depends on a healthy, vibrant physical instrument, good co-ordination and a brilliant imagination.
- Few medical practitioners and related therapists have experienced the benefits of some of the complementary and Eastern practices, and therefore do not recommend them.

Areas for the adventurous to investigate

The options available to voice scientists and student researchers are unlimited. It is a matter of being adventurous and daring to look at some of them. A few are included below:

1. Learn from sports science how to assess the body.
2. Create performance clinics where physical efficiency can be evaluated and monitored.
3. Look for possible benefits from using of a team of experts such as trainers and performance coaches. One coach/teacher cannot be expected to know, or to be able to do, everything.
4. Create projects that look at the effects of meditation, visualization, NLP and EFT™.
5. Explore the impact of Qigong, tai chi, Western mind/body techniques, and new energy healing practices based on Eastern and

Western techniques in combination with information gained from quantum physics.

6. Co-operate with several laboratories to gather statistically significant information.

7. Look for practical projects that could have immediate impact on the performer, rather than studies that confirm what is already known.

Summary: Exciting possibilities ahead

While research on the singing voice is still in its infancy and searching for direction, it is important to keep practicality in mind when choosing a research project. There are exciting things happening in sport science and in complementary therapies that offer valuable insights into singing. New areas of healing such as Quantum Touch™, EFT™, and various forms of energy healing/medicine, are interesting avenues for working with physical, mental, emotional, and psychological voice problems and for research into areas like performance anxiety. NCCAM, the National Center for Complimentary and Alternative Medicine at the NIH is devoted to research, discussion, and funding of biologically based practices, manipulative and body-based practices, Mind-Body Medicine, and the whole medical system. These interesting new possibilities are non-invasive and offer the possibility of having subjects who are comfortable rather than in awkward positions that prohibit best singing practice. All of these areas are conducive to practical and legitimate scientific research that is helpful to doctors, therapists, teachers of singing, and singers. If those who love singing are to serve the profession, it is necessary to look at the whole singer and recognize that the importance of the health of the singer and the voice are one and the same.

12   Appendices

A. Classification of singers for research

B. Study outlines for vocal anatomy

A. Classification of singers for research

Bunch, M. and Chapman, J. (2000) Reprinted from J. of Voice, Vol 14, No. 3, pp.363-369, The Voice Foundation

Categories of singers

Singers have been divided into nine categories based on proven per-formance achievement.
When a singer appears to fit two categories, always use the one above.

1. Superstar
- a singer of world-wide fame and recognition who commands the highest fees
- is supported by powerful marketing and a personal entourage
- is never out of the public eye
- commands media attention
- professional support may include teachers, coaches, repetiteurs and choreographers

2. International
- a singer who performs in the international arena
- is known to the profession and amongst the public according to specific genre or style category
- commands good fees
- agency representation
- has high levels of training and support

3. National/Big city
- a singer recognizable at the national and big city level, who usually sings in the vernacular
- has good levels of pay
- agency representation
- possibly marketing
- training and support according to what can be afforded

4. Regional/Touring (often seasonal)
- normally a young singer gaining experience
- may still be in training
- may have an agent
- rarely has marketing

5. Local community (often semi-professional)
- usually paid soloists and club singers who have sporadic engagements
- paid local prevailing rates for performance
- have variable training

6. Singing teachers
- who do not fit any of the other categories

7. Full-time students of singing (ages 18-25 in:)
- tertiary specialist training courses
- universities
- music and drama colleges

8. Amateur
- sings for pleasure (unpaid but not unrewarded)

9. Child
* pre-pubertal voice

Types of singing

Opera…. Contemporary Music Theatre……Musical Theatre……Concert/Oratorio/Recital…… Recording Artist… …Pop…..Rock…. Rap….Cabaret & Club….. Jazz….. Folk….. Gospel & Soul….. Country & Western….. Pub & Karaoke….. Church/Cathedral….. World Music….. Vocal Groups (including Barbershop)….. …Session Singer….. Busker/Street Sing

B. Classification of singers

1. Superstar
   1.1 Opera
   1.2 Contemporary Music Theatre
   1.3 Musical Theatre
   1.4 Concert/Oratorio/Recital
   1.5 Recording Artist Primarily
   1.6 Pop
   1.7 Rock
   1.8 Rap

1.9   Cabaret & Club
1.10 Jazz
1.11 Folk
1.12 Gospel & Soul
1.13 Country & Western

2. International
2.1   Opera Principal
2.2   Contemporary Music Theatre Principal
2.3   Musical Theatre Principal
2.4   Concert/Oratorio/Recital
2.5   Recording Artist Primarily
2.6   Pop
2.7   Rock
2.8   Rap
2.9   Cabaret & Club
2.10 Jazz
2.11 Folk
2.12 Gospel & Soul
2.13 Country & Western
2.14 World Music (specify type)
2.15 Vocal Groups (including Barbershop)

3. National/Big City
3.1   Opera
3.1a Major Principal
3.1b Minor Principal
3.1c Chorus
3.2   Contemporary Music Theatre
3.2a Major Principal
3.2b Minor Principal
3.2c Ensemble
3.3   Musical Theatre
3.3a Major Principal
3.3b Minor Principal
3.3c Ensemble
3.4   Concert/Oratorio/Recital
3.5   Recording Artist Primarily
3.6   Pop
3.7   Rock
3.8   Rap
3.9   Cabaret & Club

3.10   Jazz
3.11   Folk
3.12   Gospel & Soul
3.13   Country & Western
3.14   Pub & Karaoke
3.15   Church/Cathedral
3.15a   Soloist
3.15b   Professional chorister
3.15b1 Adult
3.15b2 Child
3.16   World Music
3.17   Vocal Groups (including Barbershop)
3.18   Session Singer
3.19   Busker/Street Singer
        (specify type, i.e. Opera, pop, etc.)

4. Regional/Touring

4.1   Opera
4.1a   Major Principal
4.1b   Minor Principal
4.1c   Chorus/Cover
4.2   Contemporary Music Theatre
4.2a   Major Principal
4.2b   Minor Principal
4.2c   Chorus/Cover
4.3   Musical Theatre
4.3a   Major Principal
4.3b   Minor Principal
4.3c   Ensemble/Cover
4.4   Seasonal Music Theatre/ Touring Companies/
        Summer Rep/Pantomime
4.5   Concert/Oratorio/Recital
4.6   Pop
4.7   Rock
4.8   Rap
4.9   Cabaret & Club
4.10   Jazz
4.11   Folk
4.12   Gospel & Soul
4.13   Country & Western
4.14   World Music (specify type)
4.15   Vocal Groups (including Barbershop)

5. Local community (often semi-professional)
5.1   Opera (principal parts only)
5.2   Contemporary Music Theatre
         (principal parts only)
5.3   Musical Theatre (principal parts only)
5.4   Concert/Oratorio/Recital
5.5   Church Soloist
5.6   Pop
5.7   Rock
5.8   Rap
5.9   Cabaret & Club
5.10   Jazz
5.11   Folk
5.12   Gospel & Soul
5.13   Country & Western
5.14   Pub & Karaoke
5.15   World Music
5.16   Vocal Groups (including Barbershop)
5.17   Busker/Street Singer

6. Singing teacher (who does not fit above categories)
6.1   University/Schools/Colleges
6.2   Private

7. Full-time voice student
7.1a   Post graduate specialist training courses
         (company, university, conservatoire)
7.1b   University and College
7.1c   Music and Drama School

8. Amateur (sings for pleasure)

9. Child
9.1   Opera Principal
9.2   Contemporary Music Theatre Principal
9.3   Musical Theatre Principal
9.4   Oratorio Soloist
9.5   Recording Artist
9.6   Pop
9.7   Rock
9.8   Rap
9.9   Children's Choir

Appendix B — Study Outlines for Vocal Anatomy

1. Introductory notes on anatomy

All anatomy books use *Anatomical Position* as their point of reference for describing the body. This means that there will be a universal and uniform description of where structures are located. When a person is standing, anatomical position is shown with eyes, head and toes directed forwards and the upper limbs hanging by the sides with the palms facing forwards. Note that this means the forearms and palms are considered to be anterior.

Important terminology

1.   **The planes of the body**
        (pictures of these may be found in any basic anatomy text).
        There are four imaginary planes passing through the body in the
        anatomical position

        a. Median Plane –
           passes lengthways through the mid-line of the body from
           front to back and dividing it into equal right and left halves.
        b. Sagittal Plane –
           any vertical plane passing through the body parallel to the
           Median Plane.
        c. Coronal Plane –
           any vertical plane that passes through the body at right angles to
           the median plane dividing the body into anterior and posterior
           portions (front and back).
        d. Horizontal (transverse) Plane –
           any plane that passes through the body transversely, dividing
           the body into superior and inferior portions.

2.   **Terms of relationship**
        a. Anterior (Ventral, Front) –
           nearer to the front of the body, e.g. the navel is anterior to the
           spine. Note: The anterior surface of the hand is called the
           Palmer surface and the upper area of the foot is called the
           dorsum or dorsal surface.
        b. Posterior (Dorsal, Behind) –
           nearer or on the back surface of the body, e.g. the spine is poste-
           rior to the navel. Note: The posterior surface of the hand is

called the *Dorsal* surface and the posterior surface, or sole, of the foot is called the *Plantar surface*.

   c. Superior (Cephalic, cranial, above) –

towards the head or upper part of the body, e.g. the shoulders are superior to the hips.

   d. Inferior (Caudal, below) –

towards the feet or lower part of the body, e.g. the hips are inferior to the shoulders.

   e. Medial –

towards the Median Plane or mid-line of the body, e.g. the nose is medial to the ear, the little finger is medial to the thumb.

   f. Lateral –

away from the median plane of the body, e.g. the arm is lateral to the trunk, the thumb is lateral to the little finger.

3.   **Terms of comparison are used to compare the relative position of two structures to each other.**

   a. Proximal –

nearest to the trunk or the point of origin. In describing limbs it means the most superior position, e.g. the thigh is the proximal part of the leg.

   b. Distal –

the furthermost from the trunk or the point of origin. In the case of limbs, the inferior portion.

   c. Superficial –

nearer the surface of the skin.

   d. Deep –

away or further from the surface of the skin.

2. Notes about muscle tissue

1.   Muscles can contract and relax. Contraction is caused by a nerve impulse sent from the brain. Relaxation is caused by stoppage of that impulse. A muscle can contract approximately 50% of its length and can stretch 1.6 of its length before being injured. Tension is a result of a constant „message" being sent to a muscle to contract.

2.   Muscles cross joints. That is how they create movement. The more tension a muscle has, the more tendencies there are to constrict a joint. Over a period of time this causes joint damage and injury.

3.   The area in the muscle fiber where the nerve enters is called the motor end plate. These are generally located in the middle of the muscle.

4.   A motor unit is the group of muscle fibres that one nerve (axon) serves. In large muscles like those in the thigh, the motor units are large and may contain several hundred fibres. In muscles that need to make highly refined actions—such as the fingers and muscles of the jaw, the motor unit contains only a few muscle fibres.

5.   There are special sense organs, called mechanoreceptors, located in muscle which tell a muscle when it is stretched to far or contracted too much. These are called muscle spindles. Usually they are located near the origin and insertion of muscles. They are really amazing little computers that also help to tell us where our body is in space. For example, how do I know when my arm is up in the air without looking? Other mechanoreceptors include golgi tendon organs located in the tendons of muscle. These are sensitive to stretch and keep muscles from stretching too far and from potential tearing.

6.   Problems associated with muscles:
           Strain
           Tears
           Soreness
           Scar tissue
           Infection

3. A note about muscle action and terms of movement

Muscles contract as a result of a message from the brain. When they contract the fibres shorten and appear bulkier. They release their contraction when the nervous message stops. (much like the analogy of a light being turned on and off by an electrical switch). Muscles potentially can contract 57% of their length depending upon their bony attachments; they can stretch 1.6 times their length. Unfortunately, because one rarely knows the degree of relaxation of a muscle, it is difficult to truly know how much stretch is available. Many people carry constant tension, e.g. nervous messages to muscles to contract, so determining available stretch is not easy.

For any joint movement to occur a muscle must contract. For example, bend your elbow. To do that your biceps muscle, which attaches to the humerus and upper part of your radius, contracts to cause the action. Should you now wish to straighten your arm, your triceps, located posteriorly and attached to your scapular and ulna, will contract. Those muscles on opposite sides that have opposing actions are called antagonists. Should they both try to work together, they would stiffen the arm, stabilizing it, yet rendering the arm incapable of bending or straightening properly. Sometimes such stabilization is needed, as in the hip when standing, at other times too many muscles working at once decrease flexibility and ability to respond. This kind of antagonism can happen in the throat and larynx as well. However, it is much more complicated there.

Terms connected with muscles

a.   Prime Mover –
      the muscle or group of muscles that contract to cause the movement.

b.   Antagonist –
      the opposite of prime mover. This muscle must relax if the prime mover is to do its job properly.

c.   Synergist –
      muscle or groups of muscles that work together to stabilise a joint, e.g. standing on one leg.

Terms that describe movements of joints

a. Flexion –
in general, bending or making a decreasing angle between bones
of parts of the body. Note there are   exceptions to this in the
case of the wrist and foot.

b. Extension –
straightening of a joint that is bent; the opposite movement to
flexion.

c. ABduction –
moving a part away from the mid-line.

d. ADDuction –
moving towards the mid-line.

e. Lateral Rotation –
rotation of a part of the body or a bone away from the mid-line,
e.g. turn out of the legs in the hip sockets.

f. Medial Rotation –
rotation towards the mid-line of the body.

g. Circumduction –
a combination of successive movements of flexion, abduction,
extension and adduction in such a way that the distal end of the part
being moved describes a circle (seen in arm and leg movements).

h. Supination –
turning the palm of the hand to face forwards.

i. Pronation –
turning the back of the hand to face forwards.

j. Eversion –
sole of the foot faces away from the median plane

k. Inversion –
sole of the foot faces towards the median plane.

4. Respiration

A.   **Influences on breathing patterns**
  1.   Posture and alignment
  2.   Tensions in throat, neck, chest, shoulders
  3.   Health/Disease
  4.   Mental state/emotions
  5.   Habits and learned breathing patterns

B.   **Basic mechanism of breathing (Passive-subconscious)**
  1.   Body has need for balance of CO_2 – O_2 (carbon dioxide and oxygen)
        Brain sends message to diaphragm
  2.   Diaphragm contracts and rib cage expands
  3.   Expansion of thorax creates negative pressure inside lungs and chest
  4.   The positive external air pressure causes air to enter the lungs in order to recreate balance with the internal pressure
  5.   Expiration occurs by means of the elastic recoil of the lungs, trachea and rib cage, gravity and the relaxation of the diaphragm.
        Note: the diaphragm is not an active muscle of expiration, it is simply returning to its position of relaxation after contracting for inspiration.

C.   **Active breathing** (for more strenuous activities-including singing)
  1.   **Inspiration** – Expansion of the chest
        (Ideally seen in the area of the lower ribs and back and abdomen)
        a. The main muscle of inspiration is the diaphragm
        b.   Ribs 1-6\7 increase the Anterior-Posterior dimensions of the chest
        c.   Ribs 7, 8-10 increase the Lateral dimensions of the chest
        d.   Selected muscles of inspiration
              1)   Levatores costarum
              2)   Scalenes (accessory?)
              3)   Serratus Posterior superior and inferior
              4)   Intercostals ? *(See Dynamics of the Singing Voice chapter 6)*
        e.   Other accessory muscles may be used in extremely

heavy breathing – as in sport when winded

2.   **Expiration –** Decrease in the size of the chest
a. Main muscles of expiration
    1) External and internal abdominals obliques
    2) Transversus abdominis
b. The role of subglottic pressure
    The vocal folds offer resistance during controlled
    expiration in singing, acting and in tense people.
    (It is balance that is important here)

D.   **Problems of breathing**
1.   Excessive tension
2.   Faulty patterns and habits of alignment, particularly lower
      back (lordosis)
3.   Emotional problems
4.   Pathological conditions such as:
      Emphysema, Pulmonary fibrosis, Collapsed lung
      Problems creaed by breathing toxic substances
      (polluted air, aerosols, smoke)
5.   Lesions of the spinal cord and paralysis of respiratory
      muscles
6.   Asthma
7.   Poor understanding of breathing by teachers of singing and
      musicians

5. Phonation – the larynx

Phonation

A. *Phonation* is the utterance of vocal sound. The act of making sound and speaking demands the complex co-ordination of six major parts or areas of the body:

1. The Brain – sensory and motor components
2. Muscles of Posture and Alignment – balance and efficiency
3. The Respiratory System – air supply
4. The Larynx – vibratory mechanism
5. The Pharynx – resonation and articulation
6. Articulatory structures – speech sounds, particularly consonants

B. Sound is influenced strongly by four factors:

1. Psychological – emotional state, language concepts, personal and group interaction, self-image
2. Physiological – health, sickness, genetic endowment, physical tension, and habits
3. Acoustic – reception of auditory stimuli, hearing, environment, and noise
4. Imagination and creativity

C. The mechanism of the voice requires five parts in order to function efficiently and completely:

1. Efficient, balanced alignment
2. Breath – respiratory system
3. Vocal fold vibration – larynx
4. Amplification and Resonation of the sound – Pharynx
5. Articulation – jaw, tongue, hard and soft palates, teeth, lips

Every one of the above factors are important when assessing a patient or student. This means not only listening but also looking to see what factors are affecting speech or sound. Habits and physical tensions of every kind can affect sound, particularly in the areas of alignment, the face, neck, shoulders and chest.

The Larynx

I. Anatomical aspects

A. Cartilaginous structures and bone

1. Cricoid Cartilage   (hyaline)
2. Arytenoid Cartilages – paired (hyaline – base only)
3. Thyroid cartilage   (hyaline)
4. Epiglottis   (elastic)
5. Cuneiform cartilages – paired (elastic)
6. Corniculate cartilages – paired (elastic)
7. Hyoid Bone

B. Joints

1. Crico-thyroid
2. Crico-arytenoid

C. Membranes and ligaments

1. Thyrohyoid membrane
2. Lateral thyrohyoid ligaments – from superior horn of thyroid to posterior ends of greater horn of the hyoid bone
3. Thyroepiglottic ligament
4. Cricotracheal ligament
5. Cricothyroid ligament (yellow elastic tissue)
   This ligament forms the Conus Elasticus and the Vocal Ligament
6. Quadrangular membrane – between the arytenoid cartilages and epiglottis

D. Important muscles

1. **Posterior Cricoarytenoids** – paired – adduct (open) the vocal folds
2. **Lateral Cricoarytenoids** – paired – adduct (close) the vocal folds along with the Interarytenoids
3. **Interarytenoids** – composed of the Transverse and Oblique arytenoids
4. **Cricothyoids** – paired – action stretches vocal folds and causes pitch to change

5.   **Thyroarytenoids**
    a.   The Internal thyroarytenoids form the main part of the vocal folds and are often called the Vocalis Muscles
    b.   The External thyroarytenoid are at the sides of the vocal folds

6.   **Note: The Vocal Folds „proper" are formed by:**
    a.   **the Vocal processes of the arytenoid cartilages**
    b.   **the Vocalis muscles**
    c.   **the Vocal ligament**

E.   Important anatomical landmarks

1.   Vestibular Folds – (False cords)
2.   Ventricular Folds – (True cords)
3.   Rima glottidis
4.   Sinus and saccule – located between the false and true cords
5.   Aryepiglottic folds
6.   Pharyngoepiglottic folds
7.   Piriform fossa

F.   Blood vessels

1.   **Arteries**
    a.   Laryngeal branch of Superior Thyroid
    b.   Laryngeal branch of Inferior Thyroid
2.   **Veins**
    a.   Superior laryngeal – which empties into the superior thyroid and the internal jugular
    b.   Inferior laryngeal – which empties into the inferior thyroid and then the left brachio-cephalic
3.   Lymph drainage above the vocal folds is to the deep cervical lymph nodes near the bifircation of the common carotid artery and below the vocal folds to the nodes near the upper trachea and nodes along the inferior thyroid artery.

G.   **Nerve supply from the nucleus ambiguus**

    1.   *Superior Laryngeal from the Vagus – Cranial X*
        a. Internal branch – mainly sensory
        b. External branch – motor to the cricothyroid
        (thus affects pitch)
    2.   *Recurrent laryngeal – Cranial XI*
        a. Motor to all intrinsic muscles of the larynx
        b. Sensory to larynx
    3.   Sympathetic nerves

II. Functional considerations

A.   **Extremes of registers**

    1.   Heavy – entire edges of vocal folds meet
    2.   Light – only the vocal ligaments vibrate
    3.   Note: There are many complex gradations between these extremes

B.   **Pitch**

    1.   Action of the cricothyroids
    2.   The vocal fold vibration equals the frequency of pitch

C.   **Hyperfunction** can be caused by tension and glottal shock

D.   **Hypofunction** can be caused by breathiness and lack of energy

E.   **Pathologies of the vocal folds**

    1.   Hoarseness
    2.   Laryngitis
    3.   Nodules
    4.   Bowing
    5.   Polyps
    6.   Cysts
    7.   Contact Ulcers
    8.   Malignant Lesions

6. The pharynx and soft palate

A.   **Bony landmarks**
1.   Pharyngeal tubercle – Occipital bone
2.   Styloid process – Temporal bone
       Stylohyoid ligament
3.   Lingula of the Mandible
4.   Pterygoid plates of Sphenoid bone (Medial and Lateral Plates)
5.   Palatine Bone
6.   Thyroid Cartilage (oblique line)
7.   Hyoid Bone (greater and lesser horns)

B.   **Important muscles**
1.   **Outer circular layer**
       When these muscles contract they act as a unit to squeeze food into the esophagus. During breathing and phonation these muscles need to be relaxed for optimum quality of voice.
       a.   **Superior Constrictor** – complicated origins from Pterygoid plates, ptergomandibular ligament, and lingula of mandible
       b.   **Middle Constrictor** – greater horn of hyoid bone and lower third of the stylohyoid ligament
       c.   **Inferior Constrictor** – oblique line of thyroid cartilage
       d.   **Cricopharyngeus** – cricoid cartilage –
            This muscles acts as a sphincter to keep air out of the esophagus. When we swallow, this muscle relaxes to allow food into the esophagus.
            Note: All of the constrictors insert into the posterior pharyngea raphé

2.   **Longitudinal Muscles**
       These muscles generally contract to pull the pharynx upwards during the act of swallowing.
       a.   **Stylopharyngeus** – from styloid process to superiorhorn of thyoid cartilage and pharyngeal aponeurosis. (Innervated by themotor branch of IX Glossopharyngeal Nerve)
       b.   **Palato Pharyngeus** – from palatine aponeurosis to superior horn of thyroid cartilage and pharyngeal aponeurosis
       c.   **Salpingopharyngeus** – from tympanic tube to pharyngeal wall

C.   **Layers of pharyngeal** Wall (starting from inside the mouth)

     1.   Mucosa
     2.   Pharyngobasilar fascia – lines tonsillar bed
     3.   Longitudinal muscles
     4.   Circular muscles
     5.   Pharyngeal fascia

D.   **Tonsils** (oral pharynx) lie in the tonsillar fossa between the Palatoglossus and Palatopharyngeus muscles on top of the Pharyngobasilar fascia.
Note: there are two other sets of tonsils, one located in the superior portion of the nasal pharynx (adenoids) and the other on the posterior portion of the tongue

E.   **Divisions of the pharynx**
     1.   **Nasal pharynx –** from base of skull to soft palate – Contains Eustation (tympanic) tube and Adenoids (before age of 12). Nasal resonance.
     2.   Oral Pharynx – from lower border of soft palate to mid epiglottic area. The main source of vocal resonance is this area. As it is easily changed into many shapes, the resonance and quality of voice are altered accordingly.
     3.   Laryngeal Pharynx – from mid epiglottic area to lower border of cricoid cartilage. The resonance from this area is thought to be the re-enforced resonance called the "singers formant"

F.   **Arteries**
     1.   Pharyngeal branches from the Inferior Thyroid
     2.   Middle Meningeal and Pterygoid branches from the Maxillary
     3.   Ascending Palatine and Tonsillar branches from the Facial

G.   **Nerves**
     1.   The motor supply comes from the Vagus – Cranial X with the exception of the Stylopharyngeus muscles supplied from IX,
     2.   Pharyngeal Plexus made up of Cranial X,IX
     3.   Sympathetics from the superior cervical ganglion and parasympathetics from the pterygopalatine ganglion

7. The soft palate

A. Bony Landmarks
    1. Petrosal part of temporal bone
    2. Spine of sphenoid
    3. Palatine bone
    4. Pterygoid hamulus of sphenoid
    5. Tympanic (auditory) tube

B. Muscles
    1. **Levator veli palatini** – from schaphoid fossa (pterygoid plates) of Sphenoid bone and Tympanic tube to soft palate – raises palate
    2. **Tensor palatini** – lateral to levator muscle, from Sphenoid and Tympanic tube to bony edge of palate – believed to help regulate pressure in tympanic tube
    3. **Uvula**
    4. **Palato pharyngeus** – from soft palate to pharyngeal wall and superior horns of the thyroid cartilage – raises larynx in swallowing
    5. **Palatoglossus** – from palate to back lateral portion of the tongue – action determined by whether palate or tongue is the most stable at the time

C. Arteries
    1. Palatine branches from the Maxillary
    2. Tonsillar branches from the Facial

D. Nerve supply
    1. Motor – Cranial X and XI except to Tensor Palatini which is served by motor branch of V
    2. Sensory – IX

8. The muscles of mastication

The muscles of mastication are responsible for chewing and movements of the mandible. They are some of the strongest and most used in the body. Their role in speech and singing is limited. However most speakers and singers forget this. As a result, they are among the most overused and unnecessary muscles in the act of articulating. It is known, however, that chewing actions can be used therapeutically to release jaw tension.

A.   **Bony landmarks**
       1.   Temporal Bone
       2.   Parietal Bone
       3.   Zygoma
       4.   Maxilla
       5.   Mandible
       6.   Pterygoid plates of the Sphenoid

B.   **Muscles**
       1.   **Temporalis** – arises from temporal bone and inserts on Coronoid Process of Mandible – anterior fibres raise, and posterior fibres retract Mandible (This can be observed by noting the direction of the fibres of the temporalis)
       2.   **Masseter** – arises from Zygoma and inserts on Angle of Mandible – raises mandible
       3.   **Medial Pterygoid** – complex origins from Medial side of Lateral Pterygoid Plate to insert on angle of Mandible on the INSIDE- raises and protrudes Mandible
       4.   **Lateral Pterygoid** – Complex origins from Tempero-mandibular Joint casule, sphenoid bone and Lateral Side of the Lateral Pterygoid Plate to insert in small fossa (pterygoid fovea) on the Condyle of the Mandible - causes side to side motion of the jaw
       5.   **Buccinator** – arises from Pterygomandibular Raphé and inserts on both Maxilla and Mandible – Prevents food from getting between cheeks and teeth   .
       6.   **Mylohoid** – Paired muscle forming the floor of the mouth – originates from the Mylohoid Line on the Mandible and inserts in a midline raphé.
       7.   Other related groups of muscles are the tongue and soft palate

The act of swallowing includes the following:

1. A bolus of food is formed by chewing
2. The tongue forms a seal with the hard palate
3. The bolus is propelled toward the posterior wall of the pharynx by the tongue(action of the styloglossus) and the contraction of the geniohyoid and mylohyoid.
4. As the bolus touches the posterior wall of the pharynx it triggers the sensory portion of Cranial Nerve IX, which sends a message to the brain and causes the pharyngeal muscles to contract, thus beginning the act of swallowing and peristalsis.
5. The palate is raised to prevent the bolus from entering the nose.
6. The larynx is raised and the glottis firmly closed, the bolus goes over the epiglottis and into the piriform sinuses (space between the wings of the thyroid and body of cricoid cartilages).
7. The cricopharyngeus is relaxed and open for the bolus to be pushed into the esophagus.

C. Nerve supply
1. Motor – Motor branch of Cranial N. V – Trigeminal
2. Sensory – Sensory branches of V – Trigeminal

D. Arterial supply
1. branches of the Maxillary (from External Carotid)

9. The tongue

A.   Bony landmarks
1.   Hyoid Bone – body, lesser horn, greater horn
2.   Mandible – genial tubercles (little bumps on the inner side of mandible directly in the centre)
3.   Styloid Process – Temporal Bone
4.   Hard Palate – Palatal Bones

B.   Extrinsic muscles
1.   **Genioglossus –**
fanshaped mucle with several bundles arising from genial tubercles and fanning out to form bulk of the tongue. Action depends on direction of bundles - pro trudes tongue, pulls tip downwards.
2.   **Hyoglossus –**
from body and greater horn of hyoid bone – draws base of tongue down and backwards.
3.   **Styloglossus –**
Arises from styloid process and inserts intolateral portion of tongue interlacing with the hyoglossus muscle and continuing anteriorly.
4.   **Palatoglossus –**
Arises from palatine aponeurosis and posterior edge of the hard palate and inserts into lateral sides of posterior of tongue. The Action depends on the most stable attachment – can raise back of tongue or lower palate. (Tonsil sits on this muscle).

C.   Intrinsic muscles
These muscles have no bony attachments and are located within the muscle structure of the tongue.
1.   Superior longitudinal
2.   Inferior longitudinal
3.   Transverse
4.   Vertical
Note: The actions of these muscles vary genetically.
Their movements can cause the tongue to groove or to turn over.

D. **The Frenulum** is a strong ligament at the base of the tip of the tongue and can sometimes limit protrusion and movement.

E. **Nerve supply**
1. Motor – XII Cranial – Hypoglossal
2. Sensory – IX Cranial – Glossopharyngeal serves tonsils, taste fibres to posterior 1/3 of tongue
3. Chorda tympani – Special sensory nerves that runs with Cranial VII and supplies taste to the anterior 2/3's of the tongue
4. Special note: The Ansa Cervacalis from C1,2 and 3 runs with the Hypoglossal to the Strap Muscles

10. The muscles of facial expression

Note: The muscles of expression generally insert into the skin around the face, hence their capability of creating so many different expressions.

1.   **The muscles of the scalp**
        Frontalis, Epicranius and Occipitalis – cover scalp and forehead

2.   **The muscles of the eye**
        Orbicularis occuli – surround eyelids and close them

3.   Muscles of the nose
        a.   **Procerus** – top of the nose, creates furrows
        b.   **Nasalis** – sides of the nose, flares the nostrils
        c.   **Septal** – near lips – depress nasal septum

4.   **Muscles of the lips**
        a.   **Orbicularis oris** – a sphincter surrounding the lips that draws the lips together as in a pucker or a kiss
        b.   **Risorius** – laterally from the angle of the mouth
        c.   **Zygomatic** – from the angle of the mouth to the zygoma – smiling
        d.   **Levator labii superioris** – upper lip to maxilla – sneering
        e.   **Levator labii superioris alequae nasi** – upper lip and along side the nose near angle of eye – wrinkles nose – elevates lips
        f.   **Levator anguli oris** – raises angle of the mouth – smiling
        g.   **Buccinator** – arises from mandible and maxilla and pterygo-mandibular raphe – means „trumpet“, helps us to blow
        h.   **Depressor anguli oris** – angles down from lower lip and depresses angle of the mouth
        i.   **Depressor labii inferioris** – from lower lips straight down, depresses lips
        j.   **Mentalis** – arises from mental aspect of mandible and inserts in skin of the chin – causes pouting
        k.   **Modiolus** – the bulge of muscle at the corners of the mouth where a number of muscles insert

5.   **Branches of the FACIAL ARTERY** serve the muscles of facial expression

6.   **Nerve supply**
       a.   Motor – Cranial Nerve VII – the Facial
       b.   Sensory – Cranial Nerve V – the Trigeminal, branches from the Opthalamic and Macillary divisions

7.   **Problems which involve facial muscles**

       a.   Poor dental occlusion
       b.   Speech defects
       c.   Partially deaf people will talk (move their lips) towards the good ear and over-develop one side of the lower face and lips.
       d.   Stroke
       e.   Tic doloreux

References

Abitbol J, de Brux J, et al (1989) Does a hormonal vocal cord cycle exist in women? Study of vocal premenstrual syndrome in voice performers by videostroboscopy-glottography and cytology on 38 women. J Voice 3 (2): 157–162

Abo-El-Enene N (1967) Functional anatomy of the larynx. Thesis, University of London

Ackerman R (1967) On the problem of the palate form and voice quality. Zschr Laryngol Rhinol Otol 46: 280–284

Agostoni E (1964) Action of the respiratory muscles. In: Fenn WO, Rahr H (eds) Handbook of physiology, section 3, respiration, vol 1, pp 377–386. Washington: American Physiological Society

Alexander FM (1957) Man's supreme inheritance. Kent: Integral Press

Alexander FM (1985) The use of the self. London: Gollancz

Alexander FM (1990) The Alexander technique, the resurrection of the body. The writings of FM Alexander selected by Edward Maisil. London: Thames & Hudson

Alipour-Haghighi F, Titze IR (1991) Elastic models of vocal fold tissues. J Acoust Soc Am 90 (3): 1326-1331

Andreas, S., Faulkner, C (1996) *NLP: The New Technology of Achievement.* London: Nicolas Brealey Publishing

Baken RJ, Cavallo SA (1981) Prephonatory chest wall posturing. Folia Phoniatr 33: 193–203

Balk HW (1985) The complete singer-actor: training for music theater. Minneapolis: University of Minnesota Press

Barlow W (1973) The Alexander technique. New York: Alfred A Knopf

Barlow W (1978) More talk of Alexander. London: Gallancz

Basmajian JV (1978) Muscles alive, 4th edn. Baltimore: Williams and Wilkins

Bastian R (1984) Hoarseness in singers. The NATS Bull 40 (3): 26–27

Batza EM (1971) Vocal abuse in the rock-and-roll singer. Cleve Clin Q 38: 35–38

Bellussi G, Visendaz A (1959) The problem of vocal registers in the light of the roentgenstratigraphy technique. Arch Ital Otol 60: 130–151

Berendt J (1988) The third ear: on listening to the world. Shaftsbury, Dorset: Element Books

Berendt J-E (1988) Nada Brahma: the world is sound. London: East-West Publications (UK)

Bishop B (1964) Reflex control of abdominal muscles during positive-pressure breathing. J Appl Physiol 19: 224–232

Bishop B (1968) Neural regulations of abdominal muscle contractions. Ann NY Acad Sci 155: 191–200

Bishop B (1974) Abdominal muscle activity during respiration In: Wyke B (ed) Ventilatory and phonatory control systems, pp 12–24. London: Oxford University Press

Blanton PL, Biggs NL (1968) Eighteen hundred years of controversy: the paranasal sinuses. Amer J Anat 124: 135–147

Bless D, Abbs JH (1983) Vocal fold physiology: contemporary research and clinical issues. San Diego: College-Hill Press

Boone DR, McFarlane SC (1988) The voice and voice disorders, 4th edn, pp 49–75. Englewood Cliffs: PrenticeHall

Bosma JF (1957) Deglutition: pharyngeal stage. Physiol Rev 37: 275–300

Bouhuys A (1974) Breathing – physiology, environment and lung disease. New York: Grune and Stratton

Bouhuys A (1977) The physiology of breathing. New York: Grune and Stratton

Bouhuys A, Proctor DF, Mead J (1966) Kinetic aspects of singing. J Appl Physiol 21: 483–496

Braden G (2007) The devine matrix:bridging time, space, moracles, and belief. Carlsbad: Hayhouse, Inc

Brodnitz F (1954) Voice problems of the actor and singer. J Speech Hear Dis 19: 322–326

Brodnitz F (1962) The holistic study of the voice. Q J Speech 48: 280–284

Brodnitz F (1971) Vocal rehabilitation. Rochester: American Academy of Ophthalomology

Brodnitz F (1988) Keep your voice healthy, 2nd edn. New York: Harper and Row

Brown WS jr, Hollien H (1982) Effect of menstruation on fundamental frequency. In: Lawrence V (ed) Transcripts of the Xth symposium: care of the professional voice, part I, pp 94–101. New York: The Voice Foundation

Bunch M (1976) A cephalometric study of structures of the head and neck during sustained phonation of covered and open qualities. Folia Phoniatr (Basel) 28: 321–328

Bunch MA (1977) A survey of research on covered and open voice qualities. NATS Bull 33, 3: 11–18

Bunch MA, Sonninen A (1977) Some further observations on covered and open voice qualities. NATS Bull 34, 3: 26–30

Bunch, M, Chapman J (2000) Taxonomy of singers used as subject in scientific research. J Voice 14, 3: 363-369

Bunch Dayme M (2006) The performer's voice: reaching your vocal potential. New York: WW Norton & Co

Bunch Dayme M, Vaughan C (2008) The singing book. 2nd Edition. New York: WW Norton & Co

Bushnell H (1979) Maria Malibran, a biography of the singer. The Pennsylvania State University Press

Campbell D (1984) Introduction to the musical brain. St Louis: MMB Music

Campbell D (1991) Music physician for times to come (anthol). London: Quest Books

Campbell EJM (1968) The respiratory muscles. Ann NY Acad Sci 155: 135–140

Campbell EJM, Agostoni E, Newsom Davis J (1970) The respiratory muscles: mechanics and neural control, 2nd edn. London: Lloyd-Luke

Campbell EJM, Green JH (1953) The variations in intra-abdominal pressure and the activity of the abdominal muscles during breathing; a study in man. J Physiol (London) 122: 282–298

Capra F (1990) The Tao of physics. London: Fontana Paperbacks

Cardus N (ed) (1954) Kathleen Ferrier, a memoir. London: The Quality Book Club

Carter H (1972) An investigation of the covered tone and the spread tone. Unpublished master's project, University of Southern California

Cavagna GA, Margaria A (1965) An analysis of the mechanics of phonation. J Appl Physiol 20: 301–307

Cavagna GA, Margaria R (1968) Airflow rates and efficiency changes during phonation. Ann NY Acad Sci 155: 152–164

Cavallo SA, Bacon RJ (1983) The laryngeal component of prephonatory chest wall posturing. In: Lawrence V (ed) Transcripts of the eleventh symposium: care of the professional voice, part I, pp 37–45. New York: The Voice Foundation

Chapman J (2005) Singing and teaching singing: a holistic approach to classical voice. San Diego: Plural Publishig

Chernobelskii SI (1985) Hormonal contraceptives and singers' voices. Vestn Otorinolaringol 5: 62–63

Chia M, Huang T (2005) The secret teachings of the tao te ching. Rochester: Destiny Books

Chopra D (1989) Quantum healing. London: Bantam Books

Clark FJ, von Euler C (1972) On the regulation of depth and rate of breathing. J Physiol (London) 222: 267–295

Cleveland TF (1977) Acoustic properties of voice timbre types and their influences on voice classification. J Acoust Soc Am 61: 1622–1629

Clynes M (1989) Sentics: the touch of emotions. New York: Doubleday Anchor

Clynes M (ed) (1982) Music, mind and brain: the neurophychology of music. New York: Plenum Press

Coleman RF (1987) Performance demands and the performer's vocal capabilities. J Voice 1: 209–216

Colton R (1987) The role of pitch in the discrimination of voice quality. J Voice 1 (3): 240–245

Colton R (1988) Physiological mechanisms of vocal frequency control: the role of tension. J Voice 2 (3): 208–220

Colton R, Estill J (1981) Elements of voice quality: perceptual, acoustic and physiologic aspects. In: Lass N (ed) Speech and language: advances in basic research and proactice, vol 5, pp 311–430. New York: Academic Press

Colton RH (1972) Spectral characteristics of the modal and falsetto registers. Folia Phoniatr (Basel) 24: 337–344

Colton RH (1973a) Vocal intensity in the modal and falsetto registers. Folia Phoniatr (Basel) 25: 62–70

Colton RH, Casper JK, (1990) Understanding voice problems: a physiological perspective for diagnosis and treatment, pp 310–311. Baltimore: Williams & Wilkins

Conable, B., and Conable, B (2000) What Every Musician Needs to Know About the Body: The Practical Application of Body Mapping and the Alexander Technique to Making Music. Portland, Oregon: Andover Press

Cooper M (1982) The tired speaking voice and the negative effect on the singing voice. The NATS Bull 39 (2): 11–14

Crelin E (1987) The human vocal tract: anatomy, function, development and evolution. New York: Vantage Press

Critchley MacDonald, Henson RA (1977) Music and the brain. London: Heinemann Medical Books

Crystal D (1981) Clinical linguistics (Disorders of human communication, vol 3). Wien NewYork: Springer

Cunningham L (ed) (1963) The regulation of human respiration, proceedings of Haldane Centenary Symposium. Oxford: Blackwell

Damasio AR, Damasio H (1977) Musical faculty and cerebral dominance. In: Critchley M, Henson RA (eds) Music and the brain, pp 141–155. London: Heinemann Medical Books

Damsté PH (1967) Voice change in adult women caused by virilizing agents. J Sp Dis 32: 126–132

Damsté PH (1968a) X–ray study of phonation. Folia Phoniat (Basel) 20: 65–88

Damsté PH, Hollien H, Moore P, Murry F (1968b) An x-ray study of the vocal fold length. Folia Phoniatr (Basel) 20: 349–359

Damsté PH, Lerman JW (1975) An introduction to voice pathology: functional and organic. Springfield: Charles C Thomas

Damsté, PH (1964) Virilization of the voice due to anabolic steroids. Folia Phoniatr (Basel) 16: 10–18

Darby JK, Hollien H (1977) Vocal and speech patterns of depressive patients. Folia Phoniatr (Basel) 29: 279–291

Dennison, P (1986) Brain-Gym. Ventura, California: Edu-Kinesthetics

Diamond J (1983) The life energy in music, vol I, II, and III. New York: Archaeus Press

Draper MH, Ladefoged P, Whitteridge D (1959) Respiratory muscles in speech. J Speech Hear Res 2: 16–27

Edwin R (1982) Voice and speech dynamics in the total personality. The NATS Bulletin 38 (3): 38–42

Estill J (1988) Belting and classic voice quality: some physiological differences. In: Medical problems of performing artists, pp 37–43

Faaborg-Andersen K (1957) Electromyographic investigation of intrinsic laryngeal muscles in humans. Acta Physiol Scand 41 [Suppl]: 40

Faaborg-Andersen K, Sonninen A (1959) The function of the extrinsic laryngeal muscles at different pitch. Acta Otolaryngol 51: 89–93

Faaborg-Andersen K, Vennard W (1964) Electromyography of extrinsic laryngeal muscles during phonation of different vowels. Ann Otol Rhinol Laryngol 73: 248–252

Faaborg-Andersen K, Yanagihara N, von Leden H (1967) Vocal pitch and intensity regulation. A comparative study of electrical activity in the cricothyroid muscle and the airflow rate. Arch Otolaryngol (Chicago) 85: 448–454

Feinstein, D, Eden, D, Craig, G (2005) The Promise of Energy Psychology: Revolutionary Tools for Dramatic Personal Change. New York: Tarcher/Penquin

Feldenkrais M (1980) Awareness through movement. London: Penguin Books

Fritzell B (1969) The velopharyngeal muscles in speech. An electromyographic and cineradiographic study. Acta Otolaryngol [Suppl] 250

Fritzell B, Kotby MN (1976) Observations on thyroarytenoid and palatal levator activation for speech. Folia Phoniatr (Basel) 28: 1–7

Fritzell B, Sundberg J, Strange-Ebbesen A (1982) Pitch change after stripping oedematous vocal folds. Folia Phoniatr (Basel) 34 (1): 29–32

Froeschels E (1952) Chewing method as therapy. Arch Otolaryngol 56: 427–434

Froeschels E (1967) Influence of mouth movements on the larynx. Logoped Phoniat 6: 93–94

Frommhold W (1966b) Tomographische Studien zur Funktion des menschlichen Kehlkopfes. Folia Phoniatr (Basel) 18: 81–90

Frommhold W, Hoppe G (1965a) Tomographische Studien zur Funktion des menschlichen Kehlkopfes I. Folia Phoniatr (Basel) 17: 83–91

Frommhold W, Hoppe G (1965b) Tomographische Studien zur Funktion des menschlichen Kehlkopfes II. Folia Phoniatr (Basel) 17: 161–171

Frommhold W, Hoppe G (1966a) Tomographische Studien zur Funktion des menschlichen Kehlkopfes III. Folia Phoniatr (Basel) 17: 81–90

Fry DB (1979) The physics of speech. London: Cambridge University Press

Fujimura O (ed) (1988) Vocal physiology: voice production, mechanisms and functions. New York: Raven Press

Garcia M (1894) Hints on singing (translated by Garcia B) London: Ascherberg, Hopwood and Crew

Garcia M (1971) A complete treatise on the art of singing (Excerpts translated by Paschke D). Unpublished doctoral dissertation, University of Colorado

Gattey CN (1979) Queens of song. London: Barrie and Jenkins

Gauffin J, Hammacberg B (ed) (1991) Vocal fold physiology: acoustic, perceptual and physiological aspects of voice mechanisms. London: Whurr Publishers

Gauffin J, Sundberg J (1989) Spectral correlates of glottal voice source waveform characteristics. J Speech Hear Res 32 (3): 556–565

Goldman MD, Loh L, Sears TA (1985) The respiratory activity of human levator costae muscles and its modification by posture. J Physiol (London) 362: 189–204

Gordon HW, Bogen JG (1974) Hemispheric lateralization of singing after intracarotid sodium amylobarbitone. J Neurol Neurosurg Psychiatry 37: 727

Gordon R, Shealy N (2006) Quantum touch: the power to heal, 3rd edn. Berkeley: North Atlantic Books

Gould WJ (1971) Effect of respiratory and postural mechanism upon action of the vocal cords. Folia Phoniatr (Basel) 23: 211–224

Gould WJ (1981) The pulmonary-laryngeal system. In: Stevens KN, Hirano M (eds) Vocal fold physiology, pp 23–29. Tokyo: University of Tokyo Press

Gould WJ, Lawrence V (1984) Surgical care of voice disorders. New York: Springer

Govinda A (1977) Creative meditation and multidimensional consciousness. London: Unwin Paperbacks

Govoni AF (1988) MRI of the neck and larynx. Radiol Diagn (Berlin) 29: (5) 657–667

Gramming P, Sundberg J, Akerlund L (1991) Variability of phonetograms. Folia Phoniatr (Basel) 43 (2): 79–92

Gramming P, Sundberg J, Ternstrom S, et al (1988) Relationship between changes in voice pitch and loudness. J Voice 2: 118–26

Gray S, Titze I (1988) Histologic investigation of hyperphonated canine vocal cords. Ann Otol Rhinol Laryngol 97 (4, Pt 1): 381–388

Green M, Mathieson L (2001) Voice and its disorders, 6th edn. London: Whurr Publishers

Greene B (2003) The elegant Universe. New York: WWNorton & Co

Greene HP (1924) Interpretation in song. London: Macmillan

Griffith G (1965) Artistry in singing. New York: Bella-Maria

Griffiths C, Bough D jr (1989) Neurologic diseases and their effect on voice. J Voice 3 (2): 148–156

Hakes J, Shipp T, et al (1987) Acoustic properties of straight tone, vibrato, trill and trillo. J Voice 1: 148–157

Hamel PM (1976) Through music to the self. Shaftsbury, Dorset: Element Books

Harris T, Rubin J, Howard D (1998) The voice clinic handbook. London: Whurr Publishers

Haskell J (1987) Vocal self-perception: the other side of the equation. J Voice 1 (2): 172–179

Helmholtz H (1954) On the sensations of tone. New York: Dover Pub (reissued from German edn of 1877)

Henderson WJ (1920) The art of the singer. New York: C Scribner's Sons

Heriot A (1964) The castrati in opera. New York: Da Capo Press

Hetherington J (1967) Melba. London: Faber and Faber

Hirano M (1970a) Regulatory mechanism of the singing voice. Nippon Jibiinkoka Gakkai Kaiho 73 [Suppl]: 1190–1191

Hirano M (1971b) Electromyographic studies on laryngeal adjustment at vocalization. Nippon Jibiinkoka Gakkai Kaiho 74: 1572–1579

Hirano M (1974) Morphological structure of the vocal cords as a vibrator and its variations. Folia Phoniatr (Basel) 26, 89–94

Hirano M (1977) Structure and vibratory behavior of the vocal folds. In: Sawashimu T, Cooper F (eds) Dynamic aspects of speech production, pp 13–27. Tokyo: University of Tokyo Press

Hirano M (1988) Vocal mechanisms in singing: laryngological and phoniatric aspects. J Voice 2 (1): 51–69

Hirano M, Bless D (1992) Videostroboscope. Evaluation of the larynx. London: Whurr Publishers

Hirano M, Kakita Y, Kawasaki H, Matsuo K (1982) Stereoscropic ultra high speed photography of the larynx (Author's translation). Nippon Jibiinkoka Gakkai Kaiho 85 (3): 260–264

Hirano M, Koike Y, Joyner J (1969a) Style of phonation. An electromyographic investigation of some laryngeal muscles. Arch Otolaryngol (Chicago) 89: 902–907

Hirano M, Koike Y, von Leden H (1967) The sternohyoid muscle during phonation. Electromyographic studies. Acta Otolaryngol (Stockh) 64: 500–507

Hirano M, Kurita S, Kakashima T (1981) The structure of the vocal folds. In: Stevens KN, Hirans M (eds) Vocal fold physiology, pp 33–45. Tokyo: University of Tokyo Press

Hirano M, Ohala J, Vennard W (1969b) The function of laryngeal muscles in regulating fundamental frequency and intensity of phonation. J Speech Hear Res 12: 616–628

Hirano M, Vennard W, Ohala J (1970b) Regulation of register, pitch and intensity of voice. An electromyographic investigation of intrinsic laryngeal muscles. Folia Phoniatr (Basel) 22: 1–20

Hirose H (1977) Laryngeal adjustments in consonant production. Phonetica 34: 289–294

Hirose H, Gay T (1973) Laryngeal control in vocal attack. Folia Phoniatr (Basel) 25: 203–213

Hixon T (1987) Respiratory function in speech and song. London: Taylor Francis

Hixon T (2006) Respiratory function in singing. San Diego: Plural Publishing

Hixon TJ, Langhams JJ, Smitheran J (1982) Laryngeal airway resistance during singing. In: Lawrence V (ed) Transcripts of the tenth symposium: care of the professional voice, part I, pp 60–65. New York: The Voice Foundation

Hixon TJ, Mead J, Goldman MD (1976) Dynamics of the chest wall during speech production: function of the thorax, rib cage, diaphragm and abdomen. J Speech Hear Res 19: 297–356

Hoit JD, Plassman BL, Lansing RW, Hixon TJ (1988) Abdominal muscle activity during speech production. J Appl Physiol Dec 65 (6): 2656–2664

Hollien H (1980) Vocal indicators of psychological stress. Ann NY Acad Sci 347: 47–72

Hollien H, Brown WS jr, Hollien K (1971) Vocal fold length associated with modal, falsetto and varying intensity phonations. Folia Phoniatr (Basel) 23: 66–78

Hollien H, Coleman R, Moore P (1968) Stroboscopic laminagraphy of the larynx during phonation. Acta Otolaryngol (Stockh) 65: 209–215

Hollien H, Colton RH (1969a) Four laminagraphic studies of vocal fold thickness. Folia Phoniatr (Basel) 21: 179–198

Hollien H, Damsté H, Murry T (1969b) Vocal fold length during vocal phonation. Folia Phoniatr (Basel) 21: 257–265

Howard D (2007) Voice science, acoustics, and recording. San Diego: Plural Publishing

Hunt V (1996) Infinite Mind: The science of human vibrations of consciousness. Malibu: Malibu Publishing Co

Husson R (1960) Le voix chantée. Paris: Gauthier-Villars

Jones FP (1976) Body awareness: a study of the Alexander Technique. New York: Schocken

Kandinsky W (1981) Sound (tr Elizabeth R Napier). New Haven: Yale University Press

Kimura D (1964) Left-right differences in the perception of melodies. Q J Exp Psychol 16: 355

Kirchner JA (1970) Pressman and Kelemen's physiology of the larynx. Rochester: American Academy of Ophthalmology and Otolaryngology

Klingholz F (1989) The voice of the singer in the phonetogram. Laryngol Rhinol Otol Stuttg 68 (1): 62–66

Kockritz H (1965) Language orientation. An introduction to the pronounciation of foreign languages based upon the International Phonetic Alphabet. Cincinnati: Privately published

Koike Y, Hirano M, von Leden H (1967) Vocal initiation-acoustic and aerodynamic investigations of normal subjects. Folia Phoniatr (Basel) 19: 173–182

Koyama T, Harley JE, Ogura JH (1971) Mechanics of voice production II. Regulation of pitch. Laryngoscope 81: 45–65

Koyama T, Kawasaki M, Ogura J (1969) Mechanics of voice production I. Regulation of vocal intensity. Laryngoscope 79: 337–354

La Borde G (1987) Influencing with integrity. Palo Alto, California: Syntony Publishing

Lacina O (1968) The influence of menstruation on the voice of female singers. Premenstrual laryngopathy. Folia Phoniatr (Basel) 20: 13–24

Ladefoged P (1962a) Sub-glottal activity during speech. Proc of the 4th Int Cong of Phonetica, pp 73–91. The Hague: Mouton

Ladefoged P (1975) A course in phonetics. New York: Harcourt Brace Jovanovich

Landeau M, Zuili H (1963) Vocal emision and tomograms of the larynx. NATS Bull February

Langer EJ (1997) The power fo mindful learning. Reading, Mass: Addison-Wesley

Large J (1973a) Vocal registers in singing. Proceedings of a symposium (Janua Linguarum, Series Minor, 164). The Hague: Mouton

Large J (1973b) Acoustic study of register equilization in singing. Folia Phoniatr (Basel) 25: 39–61

Large J, Iwata S (1971) Aerodynamic study of vibrato and voluntary "straight tone" pairs in singing. Folia Phoniatr (Basel) 23: 50–65

Large J, Iwata S, von Leden H (1970) The primary female register transition in singing. Aerodynamic study. Folia Phoniatr (Basel) 22: 385–396

Large J, Iwata S, von Leden H (1972) The male, operatic head register vs falsetto. Folia Phoniatr (Basel) 24: 19–29

Lawrence JL (1979) Care of the professional voice. Transcripts of the VIIIth symposium. New York: The Voice Foundation

Lawrence JL (1980) Care of the professional voice. Transcripts of the IXth symposium. New York: The Voice Foundation

Leanderon R, Sundberg J, von Euler C (1987) Breathing muscle activity and subglottal pressure dynamics in singing and speech. J Voice 3: 258–261

Leanderson R (1972) On the functional organization of facial muscles in speech. From the Departments of Otolaryngology and Clinical Neurophysiology, Karolinska Sjukhuset, Stockholm, Sweden

Leanderson R (1972) On the functional organization of facial muscles in speech. From the Departments of Otolaryngology and Clincal Neurophysiology, Karolinska Sjukhuset, Stockholm, Sweden

Leanderson R, Sundberg J (1988) Breathing for singing. J Voice 2 (1): 2–12

Leanderson R, Sundberg J, Von Euler C (1987) Role of diaphragmatic activity during singing: a study of transdiaphragmatic pressures. J Appl Physiol 62 (1): 259–270

Lethbridge P (1964) Kathleen Ferrier. London: Red Lion Lives

Lieberman P (1977) Speech physiology and acoustic phonetics: an introduction. New York: Macmillan

Lipton BH (2005) The biology of belief: unleashing the power of consciousness, matter & moracles. Santa Rose: Elite Books

Luchsinger R, Arnold GE (1965) Voice – speech – language, clinical communicology: its physiology and pathology. Belmont: Wadsworth

MacCurtain F (1981) Pharyngeal factors influencing voice quality. Dissertation, University of London

Macdonald, G (2002) Illustrated Elements of Alexander Technique. London: Element

Mackworth-Young G (1953) What happens in singing, a short manual of vocal mechanics and technique. London: Newman Neame

Marafiotti PM (1928) Caruso's method of voice production; the scientific culture of the voice. New York: D Appleton

Marchesi B (1932) The singer's catechism and creed. London: JM Dent and Sons

Marshall M (1953) The singer's manual of english diction. New York: G Schirmer

Martin F (1988) Drugs and vocal function. J Voice 2 (4): 338–344

Maue WM, Dickson DR (1971) Cartilages and ligaments of the adult human larynx. Arch Otolaryngol 94: 432–439

McCoy S (2004) Your voice: An inside view: ultimedia voice science and pedagogy. Princeton: Inside View Publishing

Miller DG (2008) Resonance in singing. Princeton: Inside View Press

Miller R (1977) English, French, German and Italian techniques of singing: a study in national tonal preference and how they relate to functional efficiency. Metuchen: The Scarecrow Press

Miller R (1986) The structure of singing: system and art in vocal technique. New York: Schirmer Books

Miller R, Schutte H (1981) The effect of tongue position on spectra in singing. The NATS Bull 37: 26–34

Minifie FD, Hixon TJ, Williams F (1973) Normal aspects of speech, hearing and language. Englewood Cliffs: Prentice-Hall

Moses P (1954) The voice of neurosis. New York: Grune and Stratton

Negus V (1965) The biology of respiration. London: E&S Lovingstone

Negus VE (1931) The mechanism of the larynx. St Louis: CV Mosby

Negus VE (1962) The comparative anatomy and physiology of the larynx. New York: Hafner

Nelson S, Blades-Zeller E (2000) Singing with Your Whole Self: The Feldenkrais Method and Voice. Rochester, New York: Inspiration Press

Newsom Davis J, Sears TA (1970) The proprioceptive reflex control of the intercostal muscles during their voluntary activation J Physiol 209: 711–738

O'Connor G (1979) The pursuit of perfection. A life of Maggie Teyte. London: Golancz

Olson N (1983) Effects of stomach acid on the larynx. Proc Am Laryngol Assoc 104: 108–112

Oschman JL (2000) Energy medicine: the scientific basis. London: Churchill Livingston

Paget R (1930) Human speech, some observations, experiments and conclusions as to the nature, origin, purpose and possible improvement of human speech. New York: Harcourt, Brace

Perkell JS (1969) Physiology of speech production: results and implications of a quantitative cineradiographic study. Cambridge, Mass: MIT Press

Perkell JS, Holmberg EB, Hillman RE (1991) A system for signal processing and data extraction from aerodynamic, acoustic and electroglottographic signals in the study of voice production. J Acoust Soc Am 89 (4, Pt 1): 1777–1781

Perkins W (1978) Mechanisms of vocal abuse. In: Weinberg B (ed) Care of the professional voice, pp 106–115. New York: The Voice Foundation

Perkins W H (1977) Speech pathology, an applied behavioral science. St Louis: CV Mosby

Perkins WH (1975) Normal vocal tone generation: detection, diagnosis and management of vocal tone generation. In: Tower D (ed) Human communication and its disorders, vol 3: the nervous system, pp 505–514. New York: Raven Press

Perkins WH, Koike Y (1969) Patterns of subglottal pressure variations during phonation. Folia Phoniatr (Basel) 21: 1–18

Perkins WH, Sawyer P (1958) Research on vocal efficiency. The NATS Bulletin 15: 4–7

Perkins WH, Yanagihara N (1968) Parameters of voice production I. Some mechanisms for the regulation of pitch. J Speech Hear Res 11: 246–267

Pert C (1997) Molecules of Emotion: Why you feel the way you feel. London: Simon & Schuster

Pleasants H (1966) The great singers. New York: Simon and Schuster

Poole JL (1989) Weight and the singing voice (Viewpoint column). Opera News 3: 4

Proctor DF (1980) Breathing, speech and song. Wien New York: Springer

Promislow, S (1999) Making the Brain Body Connection. West Vancouver: Kinetic Publishing

Ristad E (1982) A soprano on her head. Right-side-up reflections on life and other performances. Moab, Utah: Real People

Rothenberg M, Miller D, Molitor R (1988) Aerodynamic investigation of sources of vibrato. Folia Phoniatria 40: 244–260

Rousey CL (ed) (1974) Psychiatric assessment by speech and hearing behavior. Springfield: Charles C Thomas

Rubin HJ, Hirt CC (1960) The falsetto. A high speed cinematographic study. Laryngoscope 70: 1305–1324

Rubin HJ, Lecover M, Vennard W (1967) Vocal intensity subglottic pressure and air flow relationships in singers. Folia Phoniatr (Basel) 19: 393–413

Rubin JR, Sataloff RT (2006) Diagnosis and treatment of voice disorders. 3rd Edition. San Diego: Plural Publishing

Rubin W (1988) Allergic, dietary, chemical, stress, and hormonal influences in voice abnormalities. J Voice 1 (4): 378–385

Rudhyar D (1982) The magic of tone and the art of music. London: Shambhala

Russell A (1952) Anna Russell sings? New York Town Hall Recital, Phillips Recording BBL 7008

Russell G (1928) The vowel, its physiological mechanism as shown by x-rays. Columbus: The Ohio State University Press

Sanders R (2004) Biomechanical Analyses in Physical Education. In: Critical Inquiry and Problem Solving in Physical Education. Routeledge

Sataloff RT (1990) Medical problems of the aging singer. In: Abstracts, Pacific Voice Conference, San Franscisco

Sataloff RT (2006) Vocal health and pedagogy, Vol 1 and Vol II, 2nd Ed. San Diego: Plural Publishing

Sataloff, R (2005) Professional Voice: The Science and Art of Clinical Care. 3rd Edition. San Diego: Plural Publishing

Schultz-Coulon HJ (1978) The neuromuscular phonatory control system and vocal function. Acta Otolaryngol 86: 142–153

Schutte H, Miller R (1984) Breath management in repeated vocal onset. Folia Phoniatria 36: 225–232

Schutte HK (1986) Aerodynamics of phonation. Acta Otorhinolaryngol (Belg) 40 (2): 344–357

Scotto di Carlo N (1979) Perturbing effects of overarticulation in singing. J Res Sing 2: 10–27

Sears TA (1973a) Servo control of the intercostal muscles. In: de Smedt (ed) New developments in EMG and clinical neurophysiology. Basel: Karger Sears TA (1973b) The afferent regulation of learned movements. Brain Res 71: 465–473

Sears TA (1977) Some neural and mechanical aspects of singing. In: Critchley M, Henson RA (eds) Music and the brain, pp 78–94. London: Heinemann Medical Books

Sears TA (1984) Spinal integration and rhythm generation in breathing. Bull Eur Physiopathol Respir 20 (5): 399–401

Sears TA (1990) Central rhythm generation and spinal integration. Chest Mr 97 [Suppl] 3: 455–515

Sears TA, Newsom Davis J (1968) The control of respiratory muscles during voluntary breathing. Ann NY Acad Sci 155: 183–190

Seashore CE (1932) Psychology of the vibrato in voice and instrument. In: Studies in the psychology of music, vol 1. Iowa: The University Press

Seashore H (1936) An objective analysis of artistic singing. In: Studies in the psychology of music, vol 4. Iowa: The University Press

Seidner W, Schutte JK, et al (1985) Dependence of the high singing formant on pitch and vowel in different voice types. Proceedings of the Stockholm Music Acoustics Conference 1983 (SMAC 83) 46: (1) 261–268. Stockholm: Royal Swedish Academy of Music

Shipp T (1987) Vertical laryngeal position: research findings and application for singers. J Voice 1 (3): 217–219

Shipp T, Hakes J (1985) Voice frequency oscillations during vibrato, trill, and trillo. In: Lawrence V (ed) Transcripts of the fourteenth symposium: care of the professional voice, pp 72–75. New York: The Voice Foundation

Shipp T, Leanderson R, Sundberg J (1980) Some acoustic characteristics of vocal vibrato. J Res Sing 4: 18–25

Shuter R (1968) The psychology of musical ability. London: Mathews

Silverman EM, Zimmer LH (1978) Effect of the menstrual cycle on voice quality. Arch Otolaryngol 104: 7–10

Smith GA (1977) Voice analysis for the measurement of anxiety. Br J Med Psychol 50: 367–373

Smith GA, Burkland LW (1966) Dominant hemispherectomy. Science 153: 1280

Snyderman C, Weissmann J, Tabor E, Curtin H (1991) Crack cocaine burns of the larynx. Arch Otolaryngol Head Neck Surg 11 (7): 792–795

Söderström E (1979) In my own key. London: Hamish Hamilton

Sonninen A (1968) The external frame function in the control of pitch in the human voice. In: Bouhuys A (ed) Sound production in man. New York: Ann NY Acad Sci

Sonninen A (1970) Phoniatric viewpoints on hoarseness. Acta Otolaryngol 263: 68–81

Sonninen A, Damsté PH, et al (1974) Microdynamics in vocal fold vibration. Acta Otolaryngol 78: 129–134

Sonninen A, Damsté PH, Jol J, Foktrens J (1972) On vocal strain. Folia Phoniatr (Basel) 24: 321–332

Sonninen, A (1956) The role of the external laryngeal muscles in length–adjustment of the vocal cords in singing. Acta Otolaryngol [Suppl] 130

Steiner R (1983) The inner nature of music and the experience of tone (selected lectures). New York: The Anthroposophic Press

Stockhausen K (1989) Towards a cosmic music (tr T Nevill). Shaftsbury, Dorset: Element Books

Storr A (1992) Music and the Mind. New York: The Free Press

Subtelny JD, Subtelny JD (1962) Roentgenographic techniques and phonetic research. Proc of the IVth Int Cong of Phonetics, pp 129–146

Sundberg J (1977) The acoustics of the singing voice. Sci Amer 236: 82–91

Sundberg J (1983) Chest wall vibrations in singers. J Speech Hear Res 26 (3): 329–340

Sundberg J (1987) The science of the singing voice. DeKalb: Northern Illinois University Press

Sundberg J (1990) What's so special about singers? J Voice 4: 107–119

Sundberg J (1991) Subglottal pressure control during singing. J Voice 5 (4): 283–291

Sundberg J (ed) (1983) Studies of music performance, no 39. Stockholm: Royal Swedish Academy of Music

Surina I, Jagr J (1969) Contribution to electromyography of the soft palate. Bratisl Lek Listy 51: 92–94

Taylor A (1960) The contribution of the intercostal muscles to the effort of respiration in man. J Physiol 151: 390–402

Taylor JB (2008) My stroke of insight. New York: Viking

Tetrazzini L (1921) My life of song. London: Cassell and Company

Titze IR (1979) The concept of muscular isometrics for optimizing vocal intensity and efficiecy. In: Lawrence V, Weinberg B (eds) Care of the professional voice, part 1: physical factors in voice, vibrato, registers. New York: The Voice Foundation

Titze IR (1989) On the relation between subglottal pressure and fundamental frequency in phonation. J Acoust Soc Am 85: 901–906

Titze IR (1989) On the relation between subglottal pressure and fundamental frequency in phonation. J Acoust Soc Am 85 (2): 901–906

Titze IR (1989) Physiologic and acoustic differences between male and female voices. J Acoust Soc Am 85 (4): 1699–1707

Tolle E (2005) A new earth: awakening to your life's purpose. New York: Penquin

Tomatis AA (1991) The conscious ear. New York: Station Hill Press

Triplett WM (1967) An investigation concerning vowel sounds on high pitches. NATS Bull 23, 3: 6–8, 50

Van den Berg J, Vennard W, et al (1960) Voice production. The vibrating larynx. Medical research film, produced and distributed by Stichting Film en Watenschap, Utrecht

Van den Berg JW (1955b) On the role of the laryngeal ventricle in voice production. Folia Phoniatr (Basel) 7: 57–69

Van den Berg JW (1956) Physiology on physics of voice production. Acta Physiol Pharmacol Neerlandica 5: 40–55

Van den Berg JW (1957) Subglottic pressure and vibrations of the vocal folds. Folia Phoniatr (Basel) 9: 65–71

Van den Berg JW (1968a) Register problems. Ann NY Acad Sci 155: 129–134

Van den Berg JW (1968b) Sound production in isolated human larynges. Ann NY Acad Sci 155: 18–27

Vennard W (1964) An experiment to evaluate the importance of nasal resonance in singing. Folia Phoniatr (Basel) 16: 146–153

Vennard W (1967) Singing: the mechanism and technic, 4th edn. New York: Carl Fischer

Vennard W (1973) Developing voices. New York: Carl Fischer

Vennard W, Hirano M (1971) The varieties of voice production. The NATS Bull 27: 26–30

Vennard W, Hirano M, Fritzell B (1971) The extrinsic laryngeal muscles. The NATS Bull 27, 4: 22–30

Vennard W, Hirano M, Ohala J (1970) Regulation of register, pitch and intensity of voice: an electromyographic investigation of intrinsic laryngeal muscles. Folia Phoniatr (Basel) 22: 1–20

Vennard W, Hirano M, Ohala J (1971) Laryngeal synergy in singing chest, head, and falsetto. The NATS Bull 27, 1: 16–21

Vennard W, Isshiki N (1964) Coup de glotte, a misunderstood expression. The NATS Bull 20, 3: 15–18

Vennard W, von Leden H (1967) The importance of intensity modulation in the perception of a trill. Folia Phoniatr (Basel) 19: 19–26

Von Dürckheim KG (1977) Hara: the vital centre of man. London: Unwin Paperback

Von Dürckheim KG (1980) The way of transformation. London: Unwin

Von Leden PM (1961) The mechanics of the cricoarytenoid joint. Arch Otolaryngol 73: 541–550

Waengler H (1968) Some remarks and observations on the function of the soft palate. The NATS Bulletin 24: 30

Watson P, Hixon T (1987) Respiratory kinematics in classical (opera) singers. In: Hixon T (ed) Respiratory function in speech and song. London: Taylor & Francis

Watson P, Hixon T, et al (1990) Respiratory kinematics in female classical singers. J Voice: 4 (2): 120–128

Watson P, Hoit J, et al (1989) Abdominal muscle activity during classical singing. J Voice 3 (1): 24–31

Weiss DA (1950) The pubertal change of the human voice. Folia Phoniatr (Basel) 2: 126–158

Weiss DA (1951) The chewing approach in speech and voice therapy. New York: S Karger

Weiss DA (1955) The psychological relations to one's own voice. Folia Phoniatr (Basel) 7: 209–217

Wilder C (1979) Chest wall preparation for phonation in trained speakers. In: Lawrence V (ed) Care of the professional voice, part II, pp 25–32

Winckel F (1967) Music, sound and sensation. A modern exposition. New York: Dover Publications

Winckel F (1971) How to measure the effectiveness of stage singers' voices. Folia Phoniatr 23: 223–228

Wing HD (1941) A factorial study of musical tests. Br J Psychol 31: 341–355

Wise CM (1957) Applied phonetics. Englewood Cliffs: Prentice-Hall

Wyke BD (1974a) Laryngeal neuromuscular control systems in singing. Folia Phoniatr (Basel) 26: 295–306

Wyke BD (1976) Laryngeal reflex mechanisms in phonation. XVIth Int Congr of Logopedics and Phoniatrics, pp 528–537

Wyke BD (ed) (1974b) Ventilatory and phonatory control systems. London: Oxford
  University Press
Wyke BD (1979b) Neurology of the cervical spine joints. Physiotherapy 65:72-76
Wyke MA (1977) Musical ability: a neuropsychological interpretation. In: Critchley
  M, Henson RA (eds) Music and the brain, pp 156–173. London: Heinemann Medi-
  cal Books
Zemlin WP (1997) Speech and hearing science: anatomy and physiology, 4th edn,
  Englewood Cliffs: Prentice-Hall
Zukerkandl V (1973) Sound and symbol, music and the eternal world. Princeton: Prin-
  ceton University Press

Author index

Subject index

Note: Page numbers in italic indicate illustration.